ENJOY
Old Age

W · W · NORTON & COMPANY
NEW YORK · LONDON

ENJOY Old Age

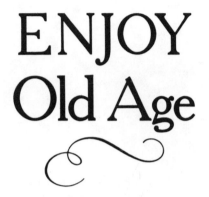

A Program of Self-Management

B. F. SKINNER
& M. E. VAUGHAN

The text of this book is composed in Avanta, with
display type set in Cheltenham Old Style. Composition and
manufacturing by The Haddon Craftsmen, Inc.
Book design by Antonina Krass.

First Edition

Library of Congress Cataloging in Publication Data
Skinner, B. F. (Burrhus Frederic), 1904–
Enjoy old age: A program of self-management
1. Old age—Psychology. 2. Aged—Psychology.
I. Vaughan, M. E. (Margaret E.) II. Title.
HQ1061.S526 1983   158'.1'0880565   83-8326

ISBN 0-393-01805-9

W. W. Norton & Company, Inc., 500 Fifth Avenue, New York, N. Y. 10110
W. W. Norton & Company Ltd., 37 Great Russell Street, London WC1B 3NU

1 2 3 4 5 6 7 8 9 0

To the memory of my father,
William Arthur Skinner
—B.F.S.

To the memory of my father,
Robert Bergh Cedergren
—M.E.V.

Acknowledgments

The authors thank Jean Kirwan Fargo for invaluable help in the preparation of the manuscript.

We have made use of a paper by the senior author, "Intellectual Self-Management in Old Age," which appeared in the *American Psychologist,* March 1983, and are grateful for permission to do so.

Contents

PREFACE 13

CHAPTER 1
Thinking about Old Age · 19

CHAPTER 2
Doing Something about Old Age · 29

CHAPTER 3
Keeping in Touch with the World · 38

CHAPTER 4
Keeping in Touch with the Past—Remembering · 49

CHAPTER 5
Thinking Clearly · 62

CHAPTER 6
Keeping Busy · 76

CHAPTER 7

Having a Good Day · 89

CHAPTER 8

Getting Along with People · 105

CHAPTER 9

Feeling Better · 116

CHAPTER 10

"A Necessary End"—The Fear of Death · 127

CHAPTER 11

Playing Old Person · 133

CHAPTER 12

A Great Performance—"The Grandeur and
Exquisiteness of Old Age" · 141

APPENDIX

A Note on the Language
in Which This Book Is Written · 155

Preface

At the annual meeting of the American Psychological Association in August 1982, in a paper called "Intellectual Self-Management in Old Age," I reviewed some of the ways in which I had tried to remain intellectually active. I was then seventy-eight. It was not a report of scientific research; it was an account of my own practices. Some of them were little more than common sense, some I had read about, but many were applications of what I had learned from a science called the experimental analysis of behavior.

At the same meeting I gave what I thought was a much more important paper, called "Why We Are Not Acting to Save the World," but the newspapers and the newsweeklies all picked up my remarks on aging. I was asked to appear on morning television shows, talk shows, and the radio. People wrote to me about their problems or those of their aging parents. Requests for copies of my paper poured in, and hundreds of copies were sent out. Evidently a large number of people were interested in doing something about old age.

A dozen publishers were soon asking me to expand the paper into a book. Unfortunately, one of the things I had recommended was that as one grew older, one should cut back on one's commitments. At that time I was finishing the last volume of my autobiography, and with the help of colleagues I had already started to write two other books. Would it be wise to add a third?

One of those colleagues was Dr. Margaret Vaughan, with whom I was writing a book-length version of my paper on why we were not acting to save the world. She had given a course in gerontology, knew the field well, and had in fact helped with my paper. She was currently writing a pamphlet that the National Institutes of Health would distribute to doctors for use in advising their older patients. She and I asked ourselves whether we could write a book about old age without infringing too much upon our other work. It appeared that we could if we made no effort to cover medical or financial problems and confined ourselves to the daily lives of active old people. This is the result.

Philosophers distinguish between knowledge by acquaintance and knowledge by description. Readers of this book will find a little of each. I have been *acquainted* with old age for a good many years, and Dr. Vaughan knows very well how it has been *described.* Much of what follows, in part from my paper on intellectual self-management, describes my own solutions to the problem of growing old. The rest, primarily the contribution of Dr. Vaughan, is a selection from the literature on aging.

There is another distinction between types of knowledge. In every field of science there are two languages. The astronomer speaks one when he tells his children that after the sun has gone down, the stars will come out; he speaks another to his colleagues. Many years ago Sir Arthur Eddington called attention to the two tables of the physicist: the writing table he uses and the same table as a collection of particles in mostly empty space. Students of behavior also speak two languages and are much more often misunderstood when they do so. Everyday English is suffused with terms that have come down to us from ancient ways of explaining human action. They cannot be used in any kind of rigorous science, but they are often effective in casual discourse.

If this book were a scientific treatise, we should

have written it in a very different way. Its contents would then have been much easier to relate to other facts about human behavior and more useful in further investigations of the problems of old age, but the book would not have served our present purpose. It would have been out of reach of millions of people who do not want to think about old age in a scientific way but still want to take steps toward enjoying it. The reader must decide whether everyday English has sufficed, and behavioral scientists must make their own translation. (They will find a few rough suggestions at the end of the book.)

—B. F. Skinner

Cambridge, Massachusetts
January 1983

ENJOY
Old Age

CHAPTER 1

Thinking about Old Age

As everyone knows, the number of old people in the world is increasing rapidly. In the United States there are now 26 million men and women over the age of 65. In 1900 there were only 3 million. At the turn of the century one could expect to live on the average only 47 years; today the figure is 70 for men and 78 for women. During the 1980s, according to the U.S. Census Bureau, there will be a 33 percent increase in the number of people over 75. Only 5 percent of those over 65 now live in nursing homes, and only 15 percent live with, and possibly receive care from, their families. Eighty percent, therefore, are living independently—either alone or with another person—and of these, 82 percent are said to be in moderate to good health. These gains are due to advances in medicine and the increased availability of medical services and to an improved standard of living.

It is good that old people are living longer and suffering less from poverty and illness than they once did, but if they are not enjoying their lives, they have not gained a great deal. By giving people more years that can be enjoyed, the practices that have helped to solve one problem have made another more crucial.

Looking toward Old Age

A good time to think about old age is when you are young, because you can then do much to improve the chances that you will enjoy it when it comes. If you were planning to spend the rest of your life in another country, you would learn as much about it as possible. You would read books about its climate, people, history, and architecture. You would talk with people who had lived there. You might even learn a bit of its language. Old age is rather like another country. You will enjoy it more if you have prepared yourself before you go.

People seldom want to know about it, however. The country of old age too often looks like a dreary wasteland. It is not described in colorful brochures at travel agencies. On the contrary, for thousands of years it has been said to be a scene of sorrow, illness, and poverty. As many people have pointed out, everyone wants to live a long time, but no one wants to be old—or to think about being old.

Young people themselves often make the prospect more dismal by viewing old age as the time when they will pay the debts they have incurred while young. They go on smoking cigarettes and defer the lung cancer to a never-never land of the future. They convert old age into a kind of dumping ground for hazardous waste.

A colorful and appealing brochure can be written. Old age is not all that bad, and planning can make it better. And young people will be more likely to plan for it if they know what can be done. An attractive future attracts, among other things, attention.

As far as health and resources are concerned, young people now often do look to the future. They exercise, eat carefully, and scrutinize the retirement plans of the jobs they choose. They are, in short, planning better for *physical* old age, but a different kind of planning is necessary for the *enjoyment* of it. That is where we hope this book will help.

The Old Age of Others

Another good time to think about old age is when you are responsible for an old person. Perhaps a parent is now living with you or near you. Perhaps you have friends who are old. You know the kinds of things that can be done if they are in poor health or short of funds, but what can you do if they are quite obviously not enjoying their lives? You may desperately want to help, if only because you would enjoy your own life more if you saw them enjoying theirs. Something more than, and different from, Medicare and Social Security is obviously needed.

You face the same problem if you are concerned about old people for other reasons. Perhaps you are a legislator who must consider laws about housing, safety, and medical care. Perhaps you are a member of the clergy who counsels old parishioners. Perhaps you are a businessman who operates a retirement village, hotel, or other facility for old people. Perhaps you are a psychotherapist, a social worker, a visiting nurse, or a member of some other helping profession. The chances are that you have looked primarily at the health and resources of old people. You can make an equally important contribution by looking at the conditions under which they are more likely to enjoy their lives.

Old Age for the Old

The prime time to think about old age, of course, is when you are old. Old age often comes as a surprise. It creeps up and catches people unawares, often because they have deliberately not watched for it. It is not the kind of thing you can learn about from early experience, because it happens only once in a lifetime. You know only what you have learned from watching old people— either in real life or in plays, in movies, and on television—or from reading about it in stories and articles. That second-hand knowledge is seldom adequate preparation for your own old age.

You have probably found it hard to call yourself old. At some point you may have begun to say "older," perhaps because that suggests only a matter of degree, and you may then have moved on to "elderly." Most of us can remember the time when we first heard someone else call us old; perhaps a time came when you gave in and said "old" too, no matter how much it hurt. But even then you may not have found it easy to understand all that the word meant or why old age should have brought so many problems.

Many people simply accept old age with all its disadvantages; they put up with its pains and losses and resign themselves to suffer in silence. Others resent it, protest it, rail against it. We are suggesting another course: Attack old age as a problem to be solved. Take all possible steps to increase the chances that you will enjoy it. We even venture to suggest that the steps you take can be among the things you enjoy. Instead of complaining of the sere, the yellow leaf, you can enjoy the autumn foliage. Instead of learning to bear the taste of bitter fruit, you can squeeze that last sweet drop of juice from the orange.

A Survey of What Follows

Chapter 2: Doing Something about Old Age. By enjoying life we mean doing the kinds of things you like to do. It has been said that if you are not enjoying your life, something must be wrong with you. More often something is wrong with the world in which you live. We acknowledge the imperfections of old age; we simply suggest that a world should be constructed in which they cause as little trouble as possible.

Chapter 3: Keeping in Touch with the World. Like every old person you have probably found that your senses are not so keen as they once were and that you move more slowly and less skillfully. Devices, such as eyeglasses, a hearing aid, and a cane, will help, of course, but too often will not help enough. You need a helpful environment—

a world with which you can keep in better touch.

Chapter 4: Keeping in Touch with the Past. Much of what you have learned is no longer as readily accessible as it once was. You forget to do things you would enjoy if you only remembered them; you are embarrassed when you forget names and fail to keep appointments. There is nothing like eyeglasses or a hearing aid for a poor memory, but there are practices that can make forgetting less frequent and possibly less costly.

Chapter 5: Thinking Clearly. You may be finding it hard to think as clearly as you once did. The basic change in the nervous system is probably the same as in forgetting and, again, there are no appropriate facilitating devices, but a more helpful environment can be arranged. Such an environment is helpful to people of any age, but particularly to the old.

Chapter 6: Keeping Busy. Retirement brings many changes. If you are lucky, you will be able to go on doing the kinds of things you have done successfully in the past. If not, you must find other things that you like to do. The alternative is boredom or depression.

Chapter 7: Having a Good Day. Old age often means a move to a smaller house or another city, and problems arise. Wherever you live, you will want to make your world as attractive and comfortable and free of annoyances as possible. You may also want to find new ways of enjoying your leisure.

Chapter 8: Getting Along with People. Growing old usually means growing physically less attractive. For that and other reasons it may be harder than before to find and keep friends, particularly young ones. Steps can be taken to make yourself better company and avoid being lonely.

Chapter 9: Feeling Better. You will not enjoy life if you are worried, discouraged, or depressed; it is much better to feel secure, successful, and cheerful. How you feel may seem to be of first importance, but what you feel depends largely upon what you do, and what you do is the thing to be changed.

Chapter 10: "A Necessary End." The feeling that most often mars old age is the fear of death. Everyone finds it hard to accept the fact that one cannot live forever. What is really to be feared is that the fear of death will bring the enjoyment of life to an untimely end.

Chapter 11: Playing Old Person. For thousands of years old people have been called selfish, stingy, crotchety, and many other unpleasant things. If you have found yourself acting in ways that confirm this view, your character is not necessarily to blame. The world in which you live is largely responsible for what you do, and in a different world you may be a different person.

Chapter 12: A Great Performance. Whitman spoke of "the grandeur and exquisiteness of old age," and like many old people you may have wondered what he was talking about. But he was not writing nonsense, and by carefully planning your life as an old person you may discover that he was not far wrong.

Our Imperfections

Not everything we say will apply to every old person. Old people come in all shapes and sizes, and what they do about old age will depend in part upon their education, their religion, their ethnic or national identity, their family, their past or present occupations, their fields of interest, and many other things. Nor will our suggestions always work. This is not a scientific treatise. It is more like friendly advice. The Prologue in Shakespeare's *Henry the Fifth*, aware of the limitations of the stage, begged the audience to "piece out our imperfections with your thoughts." We ask you to adapt what we have to say so that it applies more fittingly to your own life. In doing so you may be able to piece out some of *your* imperfections with *our* thoughts.

Boswell recorded a remark of Johnson's that has become famous: "All the arguments which are brought to represent poverty as no evil show it to be evidently a great evil. You never find people laboring to convince you that you may live very happily with a plentiful fortune." He could have said something of the sort about this book. In laboring to convince you that you can enjoy old age, are we not showing it to be a great evil? Certainly not many books are written to prove that you can be happy though young. On the contrary, as Wordsworth put it:

> Bliss was it in that dawn to be alive,
> But to be young was very heaven!

But the young have their problems, too. A great many people will tell you that they were miserable when they were young. In fact a surprisingly large number of people between the ages of fifteen and twenty-four commit suicide.

Nevertheless, it is probably easier to be happy when you are young. Browning's Rabbi Ben Ezra was unfortunately wrong; old age, "the last of life," is *not* the part "for which the first was made." We do not live in order to be old, and for young people to expect that "the best is yet to be" would be a great mistake. But what comes can be enjoyed if we simply take a little extra thought.

CHAPTER 2

Doing Something about Old Age

Psychologists have tried to find out what is different about old people. They have conducted interviews, made surveys with questionnaires and inventories, and administered tests. They have learned, for example, how old people perceive themselves, how they feel about old age, and whether they learn more slowly than younger people or forget sooner. Facts of that sort are more comprehensive than anything one can learn from knowing a few old people personally, and they have many uses. Unfortunately, they do not lead directly to practical advice, because they do not tell us *why* old people do what they do or how they can be induced to do something else.

If the enjoyment of life depends upon things

like traits of character or ways of thinking, why do those who enjoy life when they were young not enjoy it later? That question is sometimes answered by references to "development." What people do is said to depend upon how long they have been living and what stage of life they have reached. Children are particularly likely to be thought of in this way. The sentences they speak and the concepts they use are said to appear at certain times like the shoots put out by a plant. Children are also said to go through periods in which they are naturally narcissistic or negative. That may be true, but it does not suggest useful steps to be taken. To tell the parents of a problem child that they must simply wait until the child reaches a less troublesome stage is not very helpful. And to regard old age as a stage is certainly not an encouraging way to think about it. Old people cannot solve their problems simply by developing further. Becoming mature is good, but unfortunately we cannot stop at maturity. To speak of a "ripe old age" is generous; we were ripe a few years back, when it would have been better to stop developing. An effort is sometimes made to reconcile old people to old age by saying that it is natural. But there are many natural things that we escape from with satisfaction—extremes of temperature, exhausting labor, and so on. There is no "natural" reason not to enjoy old age.

An inevitable physiological process of aging does no doubt occur. Our bodies change as we grow older, and usually for the worse. But they do not do so at a fixed rate, and bodily changes are not the only ones to be taken into account. If the stages of our lives were due merely to the passage of time, we should have to find a fountain of youth to reverse the direction, but if many of our problems have other sources, we do not need to look for miracles.

Instead of counting years, we can more usefully distinguish between ages by noting what is characteristically done in each of them. Shakespeare, in *As You Like It,* begins with the infant "mewling and puking." Next comes the school child "creeping like snail / Unwillingly to school," then the lover "sighing," the soldier "seeking the bubble reputation," and in due time the older person "full of wise saws and modern instances." Eventually, of course, the stage is reached at which one "pipes / And whistles in his sound," and then comes "second childishness and mere oblivion, / Sans teeth, sans eyes, sans taste," and in the end "sans every thing."

Different people, however, do things at different chronological ages. We have all known children who were forced to behave like adults in their early years and were "old before their time," or brilliant young people who had "old heads on young shoulders." Similarly, we have all known people who have been treated like children far too long. Within the limits set by physiological aging, we act and feel young or old because of what is happening to us and what, as a result, we do. As Justice Oliver Wendell Holmes put it, "To be seventy years young is sometimes far more cheerful and hopeful than to be forty years old." And a good many people would not mind being seventy if they could act as they acted at forty.

Matters of Consequence

Enlightened developmental psychologists go beyond mere growth. They recognize that what develops is the world in which people live. People do things in different ways as they grow older because different things happen to them. The child whose words were said to appear like the shoots of a plant would never have learned to speak at all if left alone. What develops is the verbal community, as it responds in more and more complex ways to what the child says. Negativism is characteristic of a given age in a given culture if the adults in that culture tend to treat children of that age in ways that breed negativism. Freud put great emphasis on sexual development, and there are, of course, physiological sexual changes, but what people do sexually depends largely upon the world in which they live.

How people are affected by their world is the subject of the scientific analysis upon which this book is based. We shall use the analysis, so to speak, without permission, borrowing its principles but not its terms. It has much to contribute to the enjoyment of old age, and it can be discussed for our present purposes in everyday English.

An essential point is the role played by consequences. We do what we do because of what follows when we have done it. Some things "have to be done" in the sense that if we do not do them, unpleasant consequences will follow. Thus, we *have* to take our medicine or suffer aches and pains. We *have* to pay our taxes or be fined or sent to jail. We *have* to talk to people we don't like or be called unfriendly. We *have* to fill out a lot of forms or go unreimbursed for medical expenses. We learn about the consequences either from experience or from the reports of others who have in turn experienced them or been told about them.

On the other hand, there are things we "want to do" in the sense that when we do them, pleasant consequences follow. When we are hungry, we *want* to eat our dinner. We *want* to watch a favorite television show. Again, we learn about the consequences either from experience or from the reports of others.

In talking about the enjoyment of old age, we also need to speak of things we *like* or *do not like* to do. Liking depends not so much on what we do things *for* as on what happens when we are doing them. We may even like to do some of the things we *have* to do and may not like doing some of the things we *want* to do. Thus, we usually have to earn a living, but if we are lucky, we like what we do in earning it. We want to lose weight, but we do not like the exercise or the restrictive diet that losing weight demands.

It is probably impossible to arrange matters so that we shall always do what we want to do. There will be some things that have to be done. But we can convert whatever we do into the kind of thing we like, whether we want to do it or not. *And that is what we mean by "enjoying old age."* In what follows we suggest ways of changing the world of old people so that they can do more of the things they *want* to do and will more often *like* whatever they do.

Taking Our Advice

In telling you about some of the ways in which we believe that old age can be made more enjoyable, we may sound rather dictatorial. "Do this," we say, or "Don't do that." We say it, however, only in the spirit in which the waitress says "Enjoy your meal" or the taxi driver (to whom you have given a good tip) says "Have a good day." Neither we nor they are issuing orders. We are expressing wishes. The waitress is saying "Bon appétit"; the taxi driver is simply using a current form of the courteous, old-fashioned "I wish you a good day."

Even so, you may not be the kind of person who easily takes advice given in that way. Perhaps the advice you have taken in the past worked only to the advantage of those who gave it, or perhaps it was simply bad advice. If that is the case, we can only hope that something like the following will happen:

You will read the book. One or two of our suggestions will look promising. You will try them, find that, indeed, they are worth following, and continue to follow them. But something else will now have happened: You will be slightly more inclined to follow some of our other suggestions. If the results are again good, the snowball will grow. In the end you will try everything appropriate to your circumstances, and we shall have done as much as we can to help you enjoy your old age. We hope you will then agree that if we thus "meddled" in your life, at least we did so in your best interests.

In particular, we are not exhorting you to enjoy old age by an act of will. You must be *inclined* to act in enjoyable ways. Bringing that inclination about will usually require two steps. The second is the step you will most enjoy; the first brings the second within reach. For example, you will solve your problem of boredom if you become interested in something—in a different kind of music or book or field of study or sport. Certain preliminaries are needed to build such an interest, but you may not be inclined to undertake them. We hope to show that the first step—completion of the preliminaries—can be enjoyable. In other words, you are not only to enjoy old age, you are to enjoy managing your life in such a way that you enjoy it.

Enjoying life is not easy at any age if you are in poor health. If health is your problem, you will have to look elsewhere for help. We may point out, however, that just as good health is important for the enjoyment of life, so enjoyment is important for good health. It contributes to your "will to live." Moreover, much of what we say will help you to take your pills on time and in other ways follow your doctor's advice.

We do not offer a panacea. For people of any age, but particularly for the old, enjoyment is not the kind of gold that is mined in nuggets. It must be collected grain by grain. But those who mine industriously will find rich pay dirt.

~~~~~~~

CHAPTER 3

Keeping in Touch
with the World

Someone has said that if you want to know what it feels like to be old, you should smear dirt on your glasses, stuff cotton in your ears, put on heavy shoes that are too big for you, and wear gloves; then try to spend the day in a normal way. There is no denying that as we grow older our senses become less acute and our muscles weaker. The result is most conspicuous in athletes, who retire when still relatively young for just that reason. But we all find it harder and harder to do many of the things we like to do. Unlike athletes, we need not give up.

Some of the imperfections of old age can be offset in various ways. Eyeglasses and hearing aids obviously have that effect. But we can also profit from a world so designed that we can behave reasonably well in it in spite of our deficiencies. There is nothing new about helpful environments. We build them for children, providing cribs that are safer than beds, child-sized chairs and tables, and cups and spoons that can be easily held. Old people, however, need not return to childishness to profit from a world designed so that they can live in it more efficiently and hence more enjoyably.

Vision

Over half the people over sixty-five have some noticeable loss in vision. Properly fitted eyeglasses are, of course, essential, and they should stay in place without fussing. When you are reading, make sure that you are not holding your head at an uncomfortable angle in order to get a good light. A large lens mounted on a floor stand will enlarge type and can be surrounded by a helpful fluorescent ring. A large hand lens can be used as you read, and a small folding lens for pocket or purse will help at other times. With a pocket or purse flashlight, you will be able to read menus in dark restaurants and get about in dark places. Your library probably has books in large type, and some periodicals have editions printed in large type.

If your eyes adapt slowly to changes in illumination, find dark glasses that you can put on and take off easily. Wearing them in the street and taking them off just as you enter a dark store or restaurant will enable you to find your way much more easily and avoid bumping into people.

If your peripheral vision has grown weak, learn to look in new ways. In crossing streets, look farther to the right and left than you once did and look both ways to avoid being run down by a cyclist (or jogger) who is going the wrong way. Watch other people and use them as guides. If you cannot easily judge depth, learn to watch how curbs and steps change as you approach them; you can thus get a better idea of how high they are before you step down. If you have lost part of your field of vision, as in glaucoma, remember the deceptive effect of the blind spot. You are not really seeing all of what you are looking at even though you are not aware of gaps in it. When searching for something that you have dropped or lost, cover the area carefully and systematically.

It also helps to simplify your world, as blind people necessarily do. If your vision is really poor, get rid of things you don't need—in particular things that cause trouble because you can't see them easily. Clean out your cupboards and book-shelves. Small, bright-red, pressure-sensitive markers can be put on things that are especially hard to find or often needed. Whenever possible, avoid the unhappy consequences of not seeing things clearly. The drinking glasses you were given on your last wedding anniversary are beautiful—the crystal is clear, the shape pleasing. But each glass is paper-thin, with a tiny base. The slightest nudge will tip it over—and does so when you misjudge the position of the glass as you reach for it, or when your fingertips fail to report your first contact with it. A heavy drinking glass with a broad base will solve that problem.

Hearing

Roughly a third of the people over sixty show some signs of hearing loss. Hearing aids have been much more slowly accepted than eyeglasses, possibly because those who first wore them were usually particularly hard of hearing and hence were often avoided by others. Manufacturers consequently tend to emphasize concealment. The hearing aid is built into one of the temples of eyeglasses or is made small enough to fit either behind or into the ear. As a result, the volume is hard to adjust and other conveniences are sacrificed. Much can be said for the older type of hearing aid, in which microphone and amplifier were kept in a pocket and a cord ran to the ear. It had bigger batteries, so the loudness did not drop soon after the aid was turned on, and it was easy to adjust. In a noisy place it could be held close to whoever was speaking. There is no reason why such a device could not be made with bass and treble controls for adjusting it to special noise. Moreover, a conspicuous hearing aid usually induces others to speak more clearly to the person wearing it.

Fortunately, you can turn up the volume of your phonograph or radio, and headphones will protect your neighbors when you do. A small earphone can be plugged into a television set for the same purpose, and you may wish to try one in each ear by splicing the standard cord. Some sets have more elaborate attachments for the hard-of-hearing. (Beware of the temptation to enjoy too much of the once familiar level of sound produced by headphones; it can do further damage to your ears.)

Unfortunately, if you are wearing headphones you may not hear the telephone or doorbell, even when these are especially loud. A light that flashes when the telephone or doorbell rings will help. So will a pet dog who barks and dashes about when people are at the door and has been trained to do so also when the phone rings.

Adversity has its uses, and a hearing aid permits you to treat the whole world as you treat television—turning off the commercials and anything else you do not want to hear. Many years ago a cartoon by Peter Arno in *The New Yorker* showed a dowager in a box at the opera accusing her husband of having turned his hearing aid off.

Talking with other people can be made easier in various ways. Be sure it is clear to them that you do not hear well. Say so, and cup a hand behind an ear as a reminder. Speak loudly yourself. You probably hear yourself partly through bone conduction and therefore speak more softly than you suppose. Others then speak at the same level, which is too low for you. You will usually find, when speaking with friends, that if you suddenly speak more loudly, your friends will do the same.

When you do not hear well, you may often take a moment or two to understand what has been said. A remark is a puzzle, and while you are solving it you cannot make any appropriate comment. For a moment, then, you must be quite literally dumb. Worse follows if you do not succeed in solving the puzzle because by then it is too late to ask what was said. If you just say something rather vague, everyone knows that you have not understood. It is dangerous, of course, to pretend that you have heard when you have not; you may find that you have agreed to all sorts of strange things. And it is particularly bad to repeat what you think you have just heard and ask whether it is correct; your interpretation may be wide of the mark and greeted with laughter by thoughtless people. If there is a solution to that problem, perhaps it is to abandon hope. When you are sure you have heard correctly, reply quickly. When you are not sure, say "What?" at once. A companion who knows your problem and is quick to repeat a remark you appear not to have understood or have misunderstood is a great help —and should be encouraged to help.

You do best to stop trying to hear things when you are having trouble. You are probably not enjoying what is said in a television program if you are straining to hear it. Others may be enjoying it (particularly the others whose laughter has been canned), but that is no reason why you should watch. Simply do something else.

Don't go on talking with people when you are understanding very little of what they say. There are polite ways of breaking off: "I am afraid we are not broadcasting on the same wavelength." Decisive action is also needed when thoughtless people begin to speak among themselves as if you were not there. Make your withdrawal from the group clear by picking up a book or leaving the room. Deal more roughly with those who make it clear to everyone that they are talking to a deaf person.

People may forget that you are hard of hearing

and speak to you from another room or from a distance. You hear them, but not what they have said. If you then take the trouble to go and ask, they will not recognize the problem and will continue talking to you from a distance. The solution depends upon your relation with them. If you need them, go to them; if they need you, let them take the extra steps.

If you stay away from all encounters with other people because they are embarrassing or exhausting, you may find yourself leading a solitary life. A possible alternative, though not an easy one, is to do much of the talking yourself. If you have chosen the topic, all the key words will be familiar and you will be much more likely to hear what others then say. In other words, if you no longer listen well, be the speaker.

When you have trouble with eyes and ears both, problems are sometimes more than doubled. It is a common experience to be startled when you find someone near you. Thoughtful friends can learn to make their approach conspicuous, knocking on a door or approaching you only from in front. Ask them to do so. An occasional embarrassing moment cannot be avoided. The senior author of this book tells the following story:

I gave a talk at Northeastern University, and afterward the chairman of the department invited me to his home for supper with a number of students. I found myself sitting in a rather dark corner. The chairman's wife, who is Chinese, put a plate on my lap. She pointed to a rather thick dark-brown patty and said something about it, but she was gone before I was sure that I had not heard what she said. I attacked the patty with knife and fork. It had the kind of crispy crust that I had often admired in Chinese cooking, and I wondered how it was done. I had finished eating the patty before I noticed that the young woman beside me was peeling hers. I had eaten a hard-boiled egg, shell and all.

There is only one thing to do in such a case: make a joke of it.

Taste and Smell

Unless you are lucky, foods will no longer taste as they once did. They will probably be less delicious and you will be less inclined to eat them. Less saliva will flow and you may have trouble swallowing. It helps to season food a bit more and sip a drink as you eat. A dry mouth can mean trouble for your teeth, about which your dentist will advise you. If your voice begins to be affected by a dry throat, try sugar-free mints or throat pastilles.

A loss of smell is often a blessing in this increasingly polluted world, but it can be a danger too;

you may fail to smell dangerous fumes or smoke. A smoke detector will make you more secure. Aware of your reduced sensitivity, you may want to be doubly careful about odors in your own clothing and living space, which may affect your relations with other people.

Touch

The fingertips become less sensitive. You pick up a cup, misjudge the firmness of your grasp, and drop it. Heavier plates, glasses and cups, and knives and forks, will be easier to handle. You may find it harder to turn the pages of a book, especially if the paper is thin, and if so you will miss pages. Glancing at page numbers helps and can become almost automatic. And now you have an extra reason to watch the serial numbers when you separate bills fresh from the mint.

Balance

The sense organs that tell you whether you are right side up and how you are moving in space are likely to become less sensitive. In making any sudden move, you are more likely to stagger. The danger is all the greater if you cannot see well enough or move quickly enough to catch yourself as you fall. An easy solution is to move more slowly. In old age you at least have plenty of time. When out for a walk, you will find a cane helpful, even if you are not lame. (When shopping in London, ask for a walking stick; if you ask for a cane you will be referred to a store for teachers' supplies.) A light, attractive cane can be a pleasant aid. And you will feel safer and avoid accidents if you wear shoes with rough soles, and attach miniature crampons when you will be walking on icy surfaces.

Some of these suggestions are perhaps painfully obvious, but it is also obvious that old people do not always follow them and that the consequences can be painful. A single change may not mean a great difference, but with a careful husbanding of little gains, you may be surprised not only by how much better your life becomes but by how much you enjoy making it better.

the necessary steps with paper or string simply do not come back. In the same sense, words don't come back when we try to remember a poem, and notes don't come back when we try to play something from memory on a musical instrument. The steps, the words, the notes, are presumably still there, and might come back under different circumstances. People have recalled minute details of their early life under hypnosis, and almost everyone has had the experience of being reminded, for no apparent reason, of an absurdly trivial thing that happened long ago. Perhaps it could not have been recalled on demand but it was nevertheless remembered.

We can often retrieve the desired movements, words, or notes by taking a running start. We go over the steps leading up to the missing part again and again until the part appears. In that way, we reinstate more of the setting in which we made the paper hat, learned the poem, or played the piece, and so the rest comes back. Trying to recall a missing step is often described as searching in the storehouse of memory, but that figure of speech is questionable. How can we find the step if we do not know what we are looking for? We do better to think of it simply as the process of creating as best we can a situation in which we are more likely to remember.

CHAPTER 4

Keeping in Touch with the Past – Remembering

Our sense organs and muscles grow weaker with age, and so does the organ with which we use them. Changes in the nervous system presumably explain why for centuries old people have been said to be forgetful, muddled, foolish, and vague. There are no eyeglasses or wheelchairs for these impairments, but a carefully designed environment can make them less troublesome.

Forgetting is probably the most obvious symptom. What happens is clearest when we try to do something that we learned to do as a child—fold a piece of paper to form a hat or go through the steps to make the first string figure for cat's cradle. When we fail, we say "It doesn't come back to me." This is an unusually precise statement;

Forgetting a Proper Name

Proper names are especially easy to forget, and it is especially obvious that you have forgotten them. To make a proper name more likely to come back, review everything you can remember about the person or thing it refers to. Then go through the alphabet slowly and deliberately and try to pronounce the name. Sometimes you will be surprised at how quickly you can do so. At other times you will be tantalized by how very nearly you can do so, and then you may be surprised when the name pops up the next morning without warning.

Of course, you do not have time to go through the alphabet when you are introducing one person to another, so you will need other strategies. Mnemonic systems supply additional ways of getting names to come back, but they are worthwhile only when you know in advance that you will want to recall a name.

Failure to recall a name in making an introduction is embarrassing, and the embarrassment is part of the problem. It is the problem of stutterers, who are all the more likely to stutter because they have often done so with punishing consequences. We may forget a name when making an introduction simply because we are afraid we are going to forget it. Being afraid causes further trouble if we are then less likely to look at the person whose name we have forgotten. As Proust demonstrated, some very trivial feature of a situation will trigger recall, and we are more likely to forget a name if we miss some evocative detail because we are not seeing the person clearly. It often helps to make such a situation as free from unpleasant consequences as possible.

If you know in advance that you are going to have to call people by name, you can improve your chances of doing so in various ways. Before taking a friend to a club meeting, for example, review the names you will need by reading a list of the members. Or start recalling the names of people you see as soon as you arrive, before introductions must be made.

You may simply have to accept forgetfulness with good grace. You can always appeal to your age. You can please the friend whose name you have forgotten by saying that the names you forget are always the names you most want to remember. (That is true if people who are important to you make you all the more anxious not to forget.) Or recall the time you forgot your own name when a clerk asked you for it.

With the help of someone you know well, such as a husband or wife, another strategy is possible. Husbands and wives often move in different circles, and when the circles occasionally overlap, introductions may be needed. When a member of your circle approaches, shake hands, turn to your husband or wife, and say, "Of course you remember—"; thereupon your husband or wife immediately extends a hand to the new arrival and says, "Yes, of course. How are you?" Unless it is absolutely impossible that the two can have met, the new arrival will rise to the occasion. He or she will not want to seem to have forgotten a possible earlier meeting and, in any case, is probably having memory trouble too. An introduction of this kind is merely ceremonial, and nothing is lost in avoiding embarrassment. It is no more dishonest than replying to "How are you?" by saying "Fine, thank you," although you are actually miserable. You are saving the other person the labor of commiseration.

Another useful strategy is to give your own name as you extend your hand to someone you have not seen for a long time. This is an act of courtesy, and you may be rewarded by having the courtesy returned.

Forgetting How to Say Things

Of course you forget more than a word or a name. Quotations may be useful from time to time, but only if they come back in good order. You will usually be warned that you are to say grace or pledge allegiance to a temporal power, and you may be able to excuse yourself for a moment of silent rehearsal. If you forget a bit of "The Star-Spangled Banner" when singing with others, you can move your lips in a plausible fashion, but that will not serve if you have been asked to sing it solo in opening a baseball game. No good American will use written notes; nothing but a careful rehearsal will suffice.

Forgetting what you were going to say is a special case. In a conversation you wait politely until someone else finishes and then find that your own clever remark has vanished. The situation is especially embarrassing if everyone can see that you were going to say something. One solution is to keep saying it to yourself; another is to appeal to the privilege of old age and interrupt the speaker; another is to make a note (it can appear to be about what the other person is saying).

The same problem arises when *you* are speaking and digress. You finish the digression and cannot remember why you embarked upon it or where you were when you did so. The solution is simply not to digress—that is, not to interrupt yourself. A long sentence always raises that kind of problem; the last part is not likely to agree grammatically with the first because the first has passed out of reach. It is like getting up and going to another room and forgetting what you came for. Something of this sort is especially likely to happen—at any age—when you are speaking a language you do not speak well. Then it is always a mistake to embark upon a complex sentence; you do much better with simple sentences. And that is true in old age even when you are speaking your own language.

Forgetting to Do Things

Ten minutes before you leave your house for the day you hear a weather report: it will probably rain before you return. It occurs to you to take an umbrella. (The sentence means exactly what it says: the act of taking an umbrella occurs to you.) But you are not yet ready to execute it, and ten minutes later you leave without the umbrella. You can solve that kind of problem by doing as much as possible at the moment the act occurs to you. Hang the umbrella on the doorknob, or put it through the handle of your bag or briefcase, or in some other way start the process of taking it with you. The same strategy is available to remind yourself to do other things that cannot be done immediately. In the middle of the night it occurs to you that it is time to send a check to Internal Revenue. The next day you forget to send the check. Do as much as possible when it occurs to you; get out of bed and put the Revenue forms on the breakfast table.

The same problem arises when you have a good idea and then forget it. If you tend to have your ideas in the middle of the night, keep a note pad or tape recorder beside your bed. If you do not sleep alone, use a pen with a small built-in flashlight. With a pocket notebook or recorder you can preserve the things you think of at other times. The strategy is helpful to people of any age, but particularly to the old. It can make life much more effective and, hence, more enjoyable. In place of memories, memoranda.

Forgetting to Do Things at the Right Time

We seldom forget to take aspirin for a headache, but we often forget to take a pill for something as inconspicuous as high blood pressure. What is the difference? We take the aspirin for two reasons: the headache "reminds" us to take it; and when we do, we get a fairly quick result—the headache goes away. Nothing about high blood pressure or its medication has either of these effects. In general, if we are to take that kind of pill on schedule, we need two things: a reminder and a strengthening consequence.

Suppose a pill is to be taken twice a day—morning and evening. Find something else that you almost always do at those times—say, cleaning your teeth. With a rubber band, attach a small pill case to the handle of your toothbrush. As you remove it in order to use the brush, you will remember to take the pill. Unless you are an especially disorderly person, you probably do many things almost like clockwork every day—eating, combing your hair, or dressing and undressing. You can use these habitual activities as an alarm clock, to remind you when other things must be done.

For the strengthening consequence, try keeping a record of your success in remembering to do something on time. Get a calendar and a pen that makes a broad black mark. Let us say that you are to put drops in your eyes four times a day. Blacken a quarter of a day's space every time you put in a drop. At the end of the day, if you have not forgotten, the space will be solid black. As the days pass, you will be able to look at, and congratulate yourself on, a solid-black calendar. And you will probably be more likely to continue to make it black.

If your doctor advises you to walk a certain distance every day, get a pedometer—a small watch-shaped device, carried in the pocket or pinned to a garment, that miraculously records how far you have walked. Choose some distance as a goal, and on your calendar black in enough of the space for each day to indicate how close you came to reaching the goal. You may do the same with a stationary bicycle if it tells you how far you have ridden. In the long run, sustained good health and the admiration of your doctor or your friends (the practice is an excellent conversation piece, if not overworked) will make you more inclined to maintain or improve your record.

Forgetting Where You Have Put Things

"Where are my glasses?" "Where are the extra keys to the car?" There are a thousand places where you may have put them, and they will be all the harder to find if you cannot see as well as you used to. You need your glasses to find your glasses, and even when wearing them you will have trouble spotting the keys. Your fingers, too, reaching into a dark space, will not recognize objects as quickly as they once did. Learn your lesson from blind people: the only solution is "a place for everything and everything in its place."

Things are especially hard to find when you have carefully hidden them. Someone has said that no one forgets where he has buried a treasure, but many old people have wished that were true. You are going to be away for a month and have a few good things in the house that you do not want stolen. Instead of taking them to the bank, you put them in the basement or attic, skillfully hidden among old boxes, suitcases, clothing, books, and furniture. You are sure that no burglar will take the time to go through all that junk. Then, when you come back, you find yourself taking almost as much time because you cannot remember where you finally decided to put them. (Incidentally, experienced burglars know precisely where inexperienced people think no one will look.) The person who said that no one forgets where he has buried a treasure was probably thinking of pirates, but pirates knew the danger of forgetting and made maps. There would not be many stories about buried treasure if they had not done so. You, too, can solve the problem by making a map showing the location of your treasure and putting it where you can easily find it.

The problem is worse when you forget that you have hidden a treasure. You have a little more cash than you want to carry with you and do not like to leave it about the house, so you put a few bills in a book on the shelf. Years later, browsing in a secondhand bookstore, someone else finds them, looks in the front cover for your name, and sends posthumous thanks. Never forget how easy it is to forget.

Forgetting Appointments

Many of the things we enjoy—a lunch with a friend, a special program on television—must be enjoyed at a specific time of the day, week, or month. We cannot enjoy them unless we remember them, and that is the problem. A date book or calendar solves it, but only if, in turn, we remember (1) to make entries and (2) to look at them. The consistent use of a calendar can greatly contribute to the enjoyment of life, but many old people find using a calendar hard.

To make it easy, start with a large wall calendar, the kind often given away by advertisers. Hang it where you can scarcely avoid seeing it—on a wall in the bathroom, for example. Seeing it often, you are much more likely to notice the entries you have made and to think of other entries to be added. You may then find yourself looking for things to enter—not only explicit commitments but opportunities to be considered when the time comes. A glimpse of the busy hours and days that lie ahead may even lead you to plan your life more carefully. By the time you have graduated to the use of a pocket date book, you will have taken a big step toward a more enjoyable life.

A calendar will not suffice when something you want to do—watch a particular program on television, call a friend at a particular time, take frozen food out of the refrigerator an hour before putting it in the oven—must be done at a certain time of day, but a timer solves that problem. An ordinary electric alarm clock will usually do. (If you are handy, enlarge the little wheel with which you change the setting so that it is easier to turn —for example, by cementing a penny to it with a drop of epoxy.) For short periods of time and for greater accuracy use a kitchen timer. Two important consequences follow: you will enjoy the things you have not forgotten, and you will be more relaxed while waiting until it is time to enjoy them. Young people also forget, and if they develop corrective strategies while still young, they will have taken a big step toward an enjoyable old age.

CHAPTER 5

Thinking Clearly

Laurel and Hardy are looking for a hotel. Hardy sees a policeman and tells Laurel to ask him for help. Laurel goes up to the policeman and says, "Can you tell me where I can find a policeman?"

Most of us have done things just as foolish. We argue with a friend about the meaning of a word and decide to look it up in the dictionary. We go on with the conversation as we get the book down and then find ourselves looking up "dictionary." Or we stop reading and finish our coffee and then put the empty cup on the bookshelf and start for the kitchen to wash the book.

That is the kind of behavior that gives old people a reputation for being muddled and vague.

"When the age is in," Dogberry says in *Much Ado About Nothing*, "the wit is out." It is the kind of behavior that leads old people themselves to think they are losing their minds or growing senile. But people at every age may behave in that way, and sometimes with catastrophic effect. We know a recently married woman, still in her twenties, who started to put away her husband's shirts when they came home from the laundry. She removed the cardboard stiffeners, placed them carefully in his dresser drawer, and threw the shirts in the rubbish. Such actions at that age make one look to Freud. Old age is a more acceptable explanation.

You may be able to enjoy life in a muddle if you are living alone or with an understanding companion (especially one who is similarly afflicted), but if you are with others, such confusion will often be embarrassing. The essential problem seems to be the same as in forgetting. You start to do something, but the original reason grows weak and a trivial replacement can then take over. By the time Laurel has reached the policeman, he is more inclined to say "policeman" than to say "hotel." By the time you have the dictionary in your hand, "dictionary" is stronger than the word you were puzzling about. Something of the sort happens also when you are talking. You don't just forget what you were going to say;

something intervenes and you forget that you were going to say anything. As a result you ramble. "By my rambling digressions," said Franklin in his *Autobiography*, "I perceive myself to be growing old."

If you are a lawyer preparing a brief, a clergyman writing a sermon, a legislator drafting a bill, a company executive writing a report to stockholders, a scientist reporting an experiment, a member of a club preparing a book review, a concerned citizen writing a speech to give at a rally, or a writer working on a story or novel, thinking is part of your business, and a failure to think clearly can be costly. Special strategies may be needed.

A piece of sustained writing is a string of sentences. They are not arranged in the order in which they first occurred to you. (This book is not just a record of what we would have said in response to the request, "Sit down and tell me about enjoying old age.") You begin, of course, with a few things you want to say. Putting them down on paper as soon as possible will not only pin them down but keep them around to be used in subsequent thinking. They will probably fall into clusters that will begin to suggest sections of a report or chapters of a book. Some can be taken up early; others must wait until the reader has been prepared. You can arrange them and rearrange them more easily if you give them decimal numbers. Part 1 will be designated "1," with its various sections called "1.1," "1.2," and so on, and the subsections "1.11," "1.12," and so on. The numbers can be changed whenever you find a way to improve the arrangement. Relevant notes, clippings, and bits of the text can be appropriately numbered and filed. Some writers use an index card for each thought; the cards can be supplemented at any time and in the end, arranged in a logical order. An index, constructed as you go, will help you answer the question, Now where I am treating *that* point? Perhaps you were once able to do something like this in your head, although even then you would probably have done it better if you had used the rest of your body and made a record, as we have just suggested. Now, you have all the more reason to think things *out*—out in the world.

Getting into Condition to Think Clearly

You can prepare yourself to think clearly in a number of ways. Many people tend to put off this kind of serious thinking until the tag end of the day, when they are in the worst possible shape. That is a mistake. Imagine that you are a concert pianist and that tomorrow evening you will be playing a concerto with a famous symphony orchestra. How can you be sure that you will be in the best possible condition when you walk onstage? You will plan the day carefully. You will eat lightly. Perhaps you will practice, but not enough to make yourself tired. You will rest. You will find a pleasant distraction, perhaps a light novel. As a result, when you go onstage, you will be in condition to give your best performance.

Thinking clearly about a problem is as hard as playing the piano well. The same kind of preparation should be worthwhile. It is worthwhile at any age, but especially when you are old and what you have learned to say or do has become less accessible. Like the name you could remember only after a long process of recall, ideas are there, but they do not come as easily. Getting yourself ready to think does not solve the problem, but does make solving it easier.

Thinking at a slower pace helps. The slowness is not a great handicap, since old people usually have plenty of time. And learning to pace yourself as an old thinker may, in fact, give you an advantage over impetuous youth. A measured pace is advisable at any age. From kindergarten on we have probably been told to "stop and think," and we may have read in *Romeo and Juliet* that "too swift arrives as tardy as too slow."

Collecting Your Thoughts

Ideas are not hanging above you like ripe fruit on some tree of the mind, to be picked at will. They come to you in various places at various times and must be put into a form that will last until you can use them. The strategies that reduce forgetting are useful here too—a note pad or tape recorder beside your bed (if you do not sleep alone, remember the pen with a small built-in flashlight), the pocket notebook or small recorder that you carry with you as you walk, drive, or commute to work. These help you collect the ideas you will be thinking about later at your desk.

When you have put together the ideas you have collected, you will begin to see relations among them that you could not possibly see when they occurred separately. The ideas that go into a brief, a sermon, a report, a speech, an article, or a story are like the fragments of a vase found in an excavation. It would be a remarkable excavation if the fragments came into view in the order in which they fitted together, and it would be a remarkable thinker whose ideas came in the order in which they were finally expressed.

No crutches or wheelchairs are available for the verbally handicapped, but it does help to have everything needed conveniently at hand—pens,

pencils, and paper, a good typewriter or a word
processor, dictating equipment, and some way to
file and to retrieve what has been put down. A
place to think, free of distractions, is important.
Distractions are especially troublesome because
the things we are thinking about escape us so
easily. (We should have been all the more likely
to put the cup instead of the book on the bookshelf if we had been getting up to answer the
phone.) It is reassuring that these mistakes are so
often associated with absent-minded geniuses.
Absenteeism of the mind, like the absenteeism of
workers on a Monday morning in a factory, is
largely the effect of distraction.

At other times distraction can be valuable. We
often think better in the company of other people, who draw us away from our favorite themes.
We say things in a hot discussion that would not
occur to us if we were alone. Old people are at a
special disadvantage; they often lack congenial
companions. Retired teachers no longer talk to
students, retired scientists no longer discuss their
work with colleagues, retired businessmen no
longer talk with their associates. In general, old
people find themselves with companions who do
not share their interests. It will help to organize
discussions, if only in groups of two. That way,
you can exercise your mind and, most impor-
tantly, retain confidence in it.

Fear that you are not thinking clearly, like the fear of stuttering or forgetting, can make matters worse. Anything you can do to improve your thinking will therefore be matched by a gain in confidence.

Restful Thinking

Old age is rather like fatigue, except that you cannot correct it by relaxing or taking a vacation. Particularly troublesome is old age plus fatigue, and half of that can be avoided. The kind of fatigue that causes trouble is called mental, perhaps because it has so little in common with the fatigue that follows physical labor. We can be fully rested in a physical sense, yet tired of what we are doing—often to the point of being "sick of it."

We usually know when we are physically tired and need rest, but mental fatigue is costly just because we are often not aware of it. A few useful signs can tell us when to stop thinking and relax. Strange as it may seem, that idea occurred to Adolph Hitler. According to captured documents, now in the Harvard library,[1] near the end

[1]As described in an unpublished report to the Nieman Foundation by William Lederer.

of World War II Hitler asked the few remaining social scientists in Germany to find out why people made bad decisions. They reported that people did so when they were mentally fatigued. Hitler then asked for a list of the signs of mental fatigue and issued an order that any general showing such signs was to take a brief vacation. Fortunately for the world, Hitler exempted himself and continued to make bad decisions. Among the signs were some you may find helpful in spotting your own fatigue: an increased use of profanity and blasphemy, an inclination to blame others for your mistakes, putting off decisions, feeling sorry for yourself, being unwilling to take exercise or relax, and eating either too much or not enough. Another helpful sign is the tendency to use a kind of stalling: the ancient troubador was equipped with standard lines which gave him time to think of what came next, and when we are tired we fall back on phrases which have that effect. When we say "At this point it is interesting to note . . ." or "Let us now turn to another problem," we may succeed in holding the floor until we have found something worth saying, but we have not yet said it.

When fatigued we say the wrong things. Most conspicuous are the wrong words that pop out only because they rhyme with the right words or resemble them in some other way. Wrong things also include clichés, badly composed sentences, borrowed material, and the pomposities of Shakespeare's "wise saws." They flourish when we are tired, and presumably we can avoid them only by avoiding fatigue. Since many people enter old age fatigued, they are all the more in need of taking special precautions.

We recover from fatigue when we are at leisure, but the extent of the recovery depends upon what we do. We are less likely to think clearly if we spend our free time in exhausting avocations. The Greeks had a useful word—*eutrapelia*—to describe the productive use of leisure. If you are serious about solving your problems, you should carefully choose what you do when you are not solving them. Possibly you like complicated puzzles, chess, or other intellectual games. You may enjoy them, but they tire you. Give them up. Relax your standards and read detective stories or watch some of the programs on television that you once condemned as trash.

Being Creative

It is often said that those who have passed their prime have nothing new to say. Jorge Luis Borges exclaimed, "What can I do at seventy-one except plagiarize myself!" The easy things to say are the things that have already been said, either by others or by ourselves, and if what we now have to say is very much like what we have already said, we repeat. One of the disheartening experiences of the aging scholar is to discover that a point just made—so significant, so beautifully expressed— was originally made in something he or she published a long time ago.

We also tend to go on thinking in old ways just because we are committed to positions that once seemed more valid than they are now. Old scholars, scientists, philosophers, political figures, and others often go on defending views they held when they were young even though the only reason to do so is that adopting new views may appear to mean an admission of past error, a loss of prestige or position. Something of the sort holds for everyone. A change of opinion often seems like an admission of error, but the old opinion may have been right enough at the time.

To assure old people that they can continue to be creative it is customary to cite famous examples. Michelangelo lived to be 89 and was painting to the end, Verdi wrote *Falstaff* at 80, and so on. But very few people are creative in that way at any age. Francis Bacon was perhaps closer to the truth when he said, "The invention of young men is more lively than that of old, and imagination streams into their minds better." In the classic study *Age and Achievement*, [2] Harvey C. Lehman reported evidence that over the years this opinion has become increasingly valid. In the eighteenth century, he found, people tended to make their major contributions in their 40s, but in the nineteenth and twentieth centuries they have done so in their 30s. "The most creative period of life," he wrote, "has grown shorter even as life itself has grown longer."

That news would not be encouraging for old people if Lehman had not also found that in many fields there is a significant resurgence of creativity in old age. For example, his curve for the production of superior lyric poems shows a peak between ages 25 and 29 but another between 80 and 84. His curve for the production of the "most influential" books of seventy authors shows a peak between ages 35 and 43 but another between 60 and 64. Among the important pictures in the Louvre are many painted by artists in their 30s but also many painted by artists in their 70s. A great deal of chamber music was written by composers in their late 30s but a great deal also by composers in their early 70s. Philosophers

---

[2]Harvey C. Lehman, *Age and Achievement*. Princeton: Princeton University Press, 1953.

seem to have been particularly productive between ages 35 and 40 but they remain productive past 80.

Encouraging Novelty

In a sense children are original and creative because everything they do is new to them. The novel features of the world around them call for novel action. As they grow older fewer new things remain to be learned, and they begin to fall back on old routines. If the old ways work well enough, there is no reason to be original. Old people are much more likely than others to tackle a problem in old ways, and to seem less original or creative, because they have been practicing the old ways longer. But some problems cannot be solved in the old ways. (The boredom that results from a lack of variety is one of them.)

The origin of creative poems, novels, pictures, and music is like the origin of species. Just as genetic variations, possibly random, are selected by their consequences for the survival of the species, so variations in poems, novels, pictures, or musical compositions in progress are selected by their effects on the writer, artist, or composer. Creative people know (1) how to encourage variations in their work, and (2) which variations to select and which to reject. Their reputation depends upon whether their readers, viewers, or listeners agree with their selections. If a great many agree, their work is called universal.

Making Deliberate Changes

One way to be original is to make deliberate changes in the ways in which you do things. Try converting self-evident "truths" into their opposites and see what happens. If you think a given course of action must be followed, look at what will happen if it is not. If you are inclined to go in one direction, try going in another. Try especially to avoid doing things as you once learned to do them—if only to see what results. The more extravagant the variations, the more valuable may be the ones that prove worth holding onto. To vary the old Madison Avenue cliché: Run your ideas up the flagpole and see if *you* salute them.

CHAPTER 6

Keeping Busy

For many people old age begins with retirement. Since there is often some choice in the matter, it would appear that old age can be postponed. But delayed retirement is not a solution that appeals to everyone. On the contrary, most people retire as soon as they can. They are often encouraged to do so. Social Security has that effect, and old people may be told that they are holding jobs which should go to younger people who need them more. Because younger employees do not have to be paid as much, industries sometimes arrange pensions to make retirement more attractive. (In some industries old employees are encouraged to quit early and collect unemployment insurance as long as they can, with the employer making up the difference in income for that period and in subsequent pension arrangements. In thus lengthening old age, early retirement makes the problem of enjoying it all the more serious.)

Retirement is a modern idea. Until recently, as people grew older they simply did less and less of what they had always done, or turned to work that was easier. In 1870, in America, only one-quarter of the men over sixty-five were not working. A hundred years later, this figure was three-quarters. American women are "retiring" sooner too. When families were larger, parents might be in their sixties before the last child left home. Today they may be no more than forty-five. When old age starts that soon, it lasts a long time.

Those who lead an active life and like their work often think of retirement as a well-deserved rest. The pattern is established when they are young—they retire [sic] for the night; they enjoy a weekend every week; they take a vacation every year. It is easy to think of retirement from a busy life as also fitting this pattern, but rest is a restorative, and those who retire in order to rest soon find themselves anxious to get back to work—and out of a job.

Others retire as soon as possible because they have not liked their work. They have done what they had to do, and as soon as they no longer have a compelling reason to continue, they are glad to stop. They have finished the *labors* of life; retirement is an escape. But they often find that they have escaped from much that they actually liked. Their work took them out of the house, brought them into contact with other people, and took up time that now hangs heavily on their hands. Perhaps they play the golf they looked forward to, watch more television, and see more of their friends, but time remains and boredom can be painful. For most people *dolce far niente* is a recipe for a short vacation; they find that it is not "sweet to do nothing" for the rest of one's life. Very young children often have an unusual insight into what is bothering them: "I have nothing to do" is a common complaint.

The problem presumably originated thousands of years ago, when the replacement of gathering and hunting by agriculture and the domestication of animals, together with the development of improved methods of production, created substantial amounts of free time. The problem has existed ever since. It has been made worse by all labor-saving devices and practices, in spite of the gains that resulted from their invention. Throughout history affluent people have turned to gambling, violent sports, and the excessive consumption of food, alcohol, and drugs. Filling free time is also a problem of institutionalized people and people on welfare, and they seldom do any better with it than the affluent. With respect to free time, old age is like affluence and poverty. Is there a solution to this problem?

What Is Good about Work?

"All work," said Carlyle, "even cotton-spinning, is noble; work is alone noble." That contention does not carry much weight today. It is dismissed, along with other parts of the Protestant Ethic, as a device used by the rich to justify the low wages paid the poor. In its usual sense—"eminent," "highborn," or "exalted"—*noble* does seem a strange word to apply to work. Yet we see that it must refer to something when we look at those who are out of work.

There is an important distinction between the long-term consequences of work—for example, wages—and the immediate consequences. The latter are much closer to what we enjoy. To see the difference, consider a craftsman at work. He may build a piece of furniture for his own use or for sale, but that consequence follows only when the work is finished. It has little to do with the way he works or the pleasure he takes in working. Much more important to him is the way a piece of wood changes as he turns it on a lathe or carves it with a knife, or the snugness with which two pieces fit together, or the way a surface looks and feels after he has sanded, varnished, and polished it. These immediate consequences determine every move he makes and may keep him happily at work.

People write articles, stories, poems, plays, and books for the same two kinds of reasons. When a book is finished, it may sell, be admired, and bring fame, but while it is being written the important thing is how sentences look, whether they say what they were intended to say, whether they join together smoothly, and so on. Something of the sort holds also for painting pictures and composing music. The long-term effect of the completed work is one thing; what happens when the brush touches the canvas or a phrase is tested on the keyboard is another.

The difference between long-term and immediate consequences is at the heart of all games and sports. Golfers drive and putt balls in such a way that when the game is over they will have as low a score as possible or will have beaten their opponents. But whether a golfer plays well or badly, and with or without enjoyment, depends on whether the ball goes in the right or wrong direction for the right or wrong distance, and eventually on whether it drops or fails to drop into the cup. The act of controlling the movement of a ball by the movement of a club is what is enjoyed in playing golf, quite apart from winning.

Immediate consequences are the "noble" part of work, and the part most often missed when there is no work to be done. Their proper role is misunderstood when old people are said to be inactive because they "lack motivation." That phrase suggests that something is wrong with old people rather than with the world in which they live. What is lacking are the kinds of consequences that keep people busy—whether at work or play—and hence "motivated."

The depression we suffer when we can no longer do many of the pleasurable things we once did is rather like the depression we experience when we move from one city to another. Things we did in the old city can no longer be done in the new. We cannot go to the same supermarket, walk to the same neighbor's house, say hello to the same postman, take the dog for a walk on the same streets. A great many of the things we once enjoyed are no longer feasible. The resulting depression is also like missing someone who has died; everything we enjoyed doing with that person can no longer be done. When retired, we miss our job as we miss a city or an old friend.

Some Obstacles to Keeping Busy

We will find it harder to keep busy if other people, with the best of intentions, begin to do things for us. Helping really helps only those who *need* to be helped. Others are deprived of the chance to be active. (A truly compassionate God would not, contrary to the old saying, help those who help themselves. He or She would not thus deprive them of the enjoyment of achievement.) The well-meaning friend who holds our coat robs us of the chance to exercise a few seldom-used muscles. The friend who stops to give us a ride cheats us out of what remains of a healthful walk. Those who do our shopping for us convert us into stay-at-homes. Refusing help is hard because accepting it is easy and hurts no feelings, but friends who really want to help will be glad to know that we prefer to do some things ourselves.

(It is hard not to help. We watch a small boy trying to tie his shoelaces and grow jittery as he struggles. Then we tie them for him and deprive him of a chance to learn to tie shoelaces. Old people inspire the same kind of unasked-for help and suffer as much from it. Nursing homes literally hasten the death of old people by giving unneeded help. It is not always given out of compassion. Doing things for old people is simply easier, quicker, and cheaper than letting them do things for themselves.)

We cannot, of course, keep on doing all that we once did. No matter how well we may have corrected the biological imperfections of age, how many devices we use, or how well designed and helpful our environment may be, we are still likely to fail at some of the things we once did well. It is an exaggeration to say, with Bulwer-Lytton:

> In the lexicon of youth, . . .
> . . . there is no such word
> As—*fail!*

Young people do occasionally fail, but we fail more often when we are old. The natural impulse is simply to stop doing what we can no longer do successfully, but unless we find something else we shall have nothing to enjoy.

Keeping busy does not mean never resting. To rest is not to be bored. It is, rather, one of the most enjoyable things we can do—provided we need it. The nothing-to-do of boredom is nothing-you-want-to-do.

Being Busy to No Effect

Rather than find something to do, you may at times want to stop doing something you no longer enjoy, something you have gone on doing even though the old consequences seldom follow. Such behavior seems irrational, but can be explained. It occurs when consequences gradually become less frequent. A natural example is fishing in a trout stream that is slowly fished out. The fisherman waits longer and longer for the next strike. If, when he first tried the stream, he had caught as few trout as he does now, he would not have gone back. (Willy Loman, in Arthur Miller's *Death of a Salesman,* had fished out his territory.) Another example is the tragedy of the gambler who is "hooked" by early good luck and then can never stop. The simple fact is that much of what you do you learned when you were more effective. If you take a fresh look at the current consequences, you may turn to other things.

To keep busy just because you feel you should (or because you have read a book telling you that you should) is not likely to be of much help. You must get more out of what you do than an escape from feeling guilty because you are idle. Instead of trying hard to enjoy what you are doing, try hard to find something that you like better. It may take some time. You know what you like to do now, but not what you would like to do if you did it successfully.

Retiring from Retirement

The ideal way to adjust to the diminishing skill and strength of old age is to slow down and work fewer hours each day. Slowing down is often a problem. The pace at which you work is one of the things you learned when you were younger. It may no longer be right for you, but it is hard to change. Try moving very slowly for a few minutes while performing some familiar task. If you have ever seen a sloth at the zoo, take it briefly as a model. You will probably find yourself doing things in a slightly different way, which will prove helpful when you return to a more reasonable pace.

If you are forced to retire all at once, look for chances to do the same kind of work elsewhere. (Don't worry about the economy. The wealth of a nation depends upon the productivity of its citizens, and a nation is all the poorer when those who can contribute something are kept from doing so. The problem of unemployment does not need to be solved by the personal sacrifices of old people. They are among the unemployed, and they must solve their problem as the rest of the

unemployed solve it.) If you have retired because
you are no longer able to work, you may still be
able to teach others. The baseball player becomes
a manager; the football player, a coach; the businessman, a consultant. . . .

If you cannot find the kind of work you have
done in the past, try something new. It need not
be something that appeals to you at first sight.
Many people have lived unhappy lives because
they chose a field of work they thought they
would enjoy but didn't. Many have given up a
promising field before discovering that they liked
it. Perhaps your former work did not appeal to
you when you started, but you came to like it as
you became skilled in it. Look for something you
can do; the chances are, you will begin to enjoy
it as soon as you do it well. If frustration or failure
bothers you, start slowly. If you try something
new for no more than an hour or two a day under
conditions that are not too demanding, you may
be surprised at how easily you move on to longer
hours and harder work.

But don't be discouraged if you take a long
time. Remember how long you took to learn the
things you used to do. Bacon was wrong when he
said that "we learn in youth and act in age." We
must indeed learn before we act, but that is true
at any age. Old dogs have been taught many new
tricks by skillful teachers.

Things to Do

Many charitable and philanthropic organizations will be only too glad to have your help as a volunteer. You may find yourself becoming deeply involved in their objectives even though you are not particularly interested when you start. Another field which is probably open to you and in which you may slowly gain a sense of accomplishment is politics. About one-third of the voters in national elections are now over sixty-five, and they can achieve results that profoundly affect the well-being of old people—improved health care, for example, secure Social Security, and better housing. Much has recently been done to help the seriously handicapped, and much more can be done for old people, such as providing free public transportation at off-peak hours and free educational opportunities. You can work for these changes in a modest way by writing letters to editors or congressmen. You can support candidates who show some interest. You can make telephone calls at election time, address envelopes, canvass house to house, according to your ability and knowledge. The organized political power of the elderly will grow every year, and you may want to become a part of it. By doing so, you will gain in two ways: you will keep busy and you will enjoy the changes you help to bring about.

You can organize or join a local group that meets for pleasure or mutual advice on the problems of aging. You can also join and promote a national organization, such as the American Association of Retired Persons. An international organization to improve the lot of old people throughout the world may be not too far in the future. You can actively support candidates who sponsor or support legislation improving the lot of old people with respect to Social Security, inflation, health insurance, and housing.

Of all the problems of old age, keeping busy probably profits most from early planning. Instead of looking forward to retirement as a yearned-for rest or an escape from hard labor, make sure that you know what it will actually mean. When choosing an occupation, consider whether it will eventually permit you to taper off instead of coming to an abrupt stop. Taking into account the changes that old age will demand is easier in choosing an avocation than in choosing a vocation. If you have already made your choice, chances are you can still alter it to help yourself remain profitably active when you are old.

CHAPTER 7

Having a Good Day

Old age usually means changes in where and how we live. Perhaps we move into a smaller house, perhaps to the country or to a warmer climate, nearer to (or farther from) our children, closer to things we especially enjoy, or to a less expensive area. Deciding whether to move is much like deciding whether to retire: we know more about our life before moving than about what it will be like afterward. What new friends will we make? How many of the things we now enjoy will we have to give up? The decision can have distressing consequences. An old couple moves bravely into a new world, secure in the fact that they have each other, and soon the surviving member finds himself, or more likely herself, very much alone.

Wherever we live, we may find ourselves more confined to quarters. Retirement has stripped away reasons for getting out of the house, and moving about is harder. Something needs to be done to make staying at home enjoyable.

A Pleasant Living Space

Wherever you live, a sweeping simplification may be worthwhile. Moving usually makes such a simplification easy, but if you decide to stay in the same house, deliberate action may be needed. G. Stanley Hall, a psychologist who wrote a book about old age,[1] said that when he retired he went through his house, from the attic down, and got rid of everything that he did not want. He called this process "getting rid of waste material." The sheer care of a house can become a burden. You may begin to understand what Thoreau meant when he said that a man does not own a house, the house owns the man. If you can't move into a smaller house, you can at least simplify the one you have.

It may be time to give many things away—

[1]G. Stanley Hall, *Senescence*. New York: D. Appleton and Co., 1922.

unneeded things to friends or charities (especially charities to which contributions are tax deductible!) and special things to the special people to whom you were going to leave them. (If you have had lots of storage space, you may find that you have bequeathed things to yourself—that birthday present that was put away because it was not useful at the time but would have been just the thing during the past five years.)

Variety

Shakespeare said of Cleopatra, "Age cannot wither her, nor custom stale / Her infinite variety." She did not live long enough to give age a chance, but it has had its chance with you. You have probably suffered a bit of withering, but much of the staling could have been prevented. Custom is indeed the villain. It stales our lives at all ages. We tend to do what we are accustomed to do because we have done it successfully, but we suffer from the sameness.

Unless a house has been very skillfully designed and decorated, it becomes monotonous. It looks the same from day to day. The lack of variety may be a matter of carelessness. You do not play the same piece of music day in and day out, why should you have the same pictures on your walls year in and year out? You may have put them there to be looked at, but unless you are lucky you have long since stopped looking. Why put pictures on the wall at all unless you enjoy looking at them?

If you want to rediscover the enjoyment of pictures, here is an experiment worth trying. Books of excellent reproductions are often sold at large discounts. Choose one you like and take it apart. Put one page where you will occasionally see it during the day—propped up on your dining table, for example. Change it every day or week. If you discover, as you may, that each picture becomes increasingly worth looking at, you may consider buying larger ones for your walls and changing them frequently. Of course, you can easily change the music you listen to. A good radio receiver or a record player takes care of that.

There is a reason why old people find it especially hard to learn new ways of living. We continue to speak the same language as long as we are understood. When we move to a country where a different language is spoken, we must find others who speak our language or learn a new one. Similarly, we go on wearing the same kinds of clothes, living in the same kinds of quarters, talking about and doing the same kinds of things. When we move into old age and can no longer do many of them well, we must remain with other old people similarly afflicted or learn new ways of living. But just as we learned a first language more easily because we had no other language to fall back on, so we learned our first style of living more easily because we had no other style to turn to. The young must choose between something new and nothing, but old people who try something new and fail can all too easily go back to old ways.

Freedom from Annoyances

You will be more likely to enjoy old age if you can escape from minor annoyances. The point would be too obvious to mention if annoyances did not creep up so slowly that they often go unnoticed. You become desensitized. A mattress slowly changes its shape, and the way you lie on it grows less and less comfortable. To accept the discomfort without complaint is perhaps a satisfactory adjustment, but a new mattress, better designed for your needs, can make a great difference. If your favorite chair no longer fits you as it once did, a new chair can be a delight. As your vision changes, concentrated bright light may become painful. Candlelight will lose its nostalgic power and should be given up. A reading light free of glare can be a pleasant surprise.

Sudden demands on your strength are not good exercise. Doors and drawers should not stick. Carrying a heavy bag or briefcase can mean sore joints unless you add a shoulder strap. If convenient, use a small cart when you go shopping. At home, put the things you most often use within easy reach. If you have a garage, install a door opener. If you must clear away snow, use a small shovel and work very slowly, or invest in a snow blower.

Older people often need a warmer room, and any younger people they are living with may suffer. One answer is heavier clothing. New kinds of thermal underwear are worth trying. An electric blanket solves the problem at night, and you can use an electric heating pad during the day if your feet get cold when you are sitting in a chair. This is shopworn advice, but it is surprising how often it is not taken.

You do not need to move to Florida or California to change your style of dress. If there are clothes and shoes more comfortable and practical than the ones you have always worn, why not change?

Noise and pollution are increasingly serious problems. Many people simply get used to them, and that is perhaps one solution. Another is to move to the suburbs or country, but that is expensive. There are cheaper solutions. Earplugs (pieces of soft, cottony wax available at drugstores) will suppress noise from the street or the neighbor's radio or television. Air fresheners will mask, if they do not remove, unpleasant odors, and a small activated-charcoal filter will quickly give you a roomful of clean and odorless air. You may not want the manufacturers of soap, furniture polish, and cleaning fluids to determine the way your home smells. In the old days, when bad odors were largely due to poor sanitary facilities, people turned to strong perfumes and incense. You will probably survive criticism if you solve your problem in the same way.

Security

Injuries interfere with the enjoyment of life, and they do so more often when we are old because we suffer more of them. Weakened muscles and poor vision combine to increase the danger that we will fall and fail to catch ourselves when we do. We are not so likely as we once were to see the bicycle coming the wrong way as we cross a street, and we are not so likely to hear a warning call. The ritual of stop, look, and listen helps. We would have learned to look or listen when we were young if we had been born with defective vision or hearing, and it is not too late to learn now.

A useful strategy is to improve the safety of the space in which you live. Make sure that all rugs have rubber undercoatings and that there are no electric cords to trip over. Chairs should be easy to get into and out of. If you tend to fall out of bed, as some old people do, have a rail attached. Be sure all steps have railings. A rail clamped to the side of the bathtub may be literally a lifesaver. Step into and out of the tub in precisely the same way every time, like a ballet dancer practicing a difficult *pas*, while holding on to the shower-curtain rail if it is strong and within easy reach. For many decades you have done things in ways that were safe enough, but it is time to learn new ways.

You will enjoy life more if you feel secure in your home. To do so, make it secure. A large bolt on a door is reassuring. Window locks are easily installed. If you are likely to need help in an emergency, omit the bolt and leave an extra key to a standard lock with a trusted person. An easy way to call for help is essential.

A really secure home will contribute to a good night's sleep, not to mention good health. If you are afraid that you will not hear an intruder when asleep, install a burglar alarm. Besides frightening the intruder, it will awaken you instantly. Alarms are inexpensive and can be installed in such a way that you can turn them off before getting out of bed. A dog, of a size appropriate to the size of your home, may be worth the trouble of caring for it.

If you are afraid of being mugged in the streets, follow the usual advice: Walk only on lighted streets, preferably with companions, and keep away from doorways. Carry with you as few as possible of the things you do not want to lose. If your bag or briefcase is snatched, let it go rather than risk a dislocated elbow. Remember that the mugger has the advantage; give in if you want to live to be mugged another day. Your police department may have other suggestions about how to protect yourself in your area.

Programming Your Life

With retirement the schedule of your daily life may fall apart. If you live alone, you may be tempted to get up only when you please, stay in your pajamas all day, and eat whenever you are hungry. Weekends are just more weekdays. If you are living with another person, order may emerge as you adjust your schedules, but people can fall into disorder *à deux*.

There is much to be said for a fairly strict daily routine. It can have a good effect on your health. People who are continuously moving about to different parts of the world usually suffer from the disruption of their schedules. With a good routine you will not need to make decisions about what is to be done and when, and you will not so often put off enjoyable activities until it is too late. Some old people hold to the schedules they followed when young, but others need to plan anew. We have a friend who never leaves his bedroom in the morning until he has made his bed and another who never has breakfast before she has ridden the prescribed distance on her stationary bicycle. These strategies save the trouble of making fresh, and usually repeated, resolutions.

A favorite television program pins down a given hour of the day, and periods of work, exercise, and leisure can be built around it. If you have read the detective stories of Rex Stout, you may take Nero Wolfe for your model: no matter how pressing the case upon which he is working, he spends an appointed hour with his orchids. You may find it helpful to have appointed hours for meditation, reading, letter writing, taking care of household matters, and reviewing your success in managing your life (exercising on schedule, eating the right things, and following the doctor's advice—and possibly our advice, too).

Diet and Exercise

Proper diet and exercise contribute to a long and healthy life and hence to an enjoyable one. Your doctor can best tell you what you should eat and how much exercise you should take, but unfortunately knowing what you should do does not necessarily mean that you will do it. Keeping a record can help. Set goals and fill in part of a day's space in a calendar to show how close you come to reaching them day by day. Find a place where you enjoy walking, or give yourself some other reason for getting out. We know a woman who buys only enough groceries for that day's dinner. She is thus "forced" out of the house even when she does not feel like going; pleasant things happen on the way, and when she returns she is always glad that she went.

Leisure

What we do, whether in the space we have now made as pleasant and comfortable as possible or away from it, is especially important for the enjoyment of life. Indeed, it has been said that happiness in the second forty years of life depends more upon how we use our leisure than upon anything else.

Old people have more time to do things, but it is often hard to find the things to do. There is little to be said for just killing time. Thoreau claimed that we cannot kill time without injuring eternity, and that may or may not be true, but certainly we cannot do so without shortening the time that remains for us to enjoy. We need to find ways to *fill* time. Much depends, of course, upon finances. But it is consoling to reflect that the leisure classes have never solved the problem very successfully, either—they do more of the things people do in their free time, but have not become conspicuously happier. Many things can be done with limited resources.

If you once played a musical instrument, or wrote poems or stories, or painted pictures, or collected stamps, try doing so again. Many local libraries contain more than books; they are much richer in things to do than people realize. A radio solves the problem of finding music to listen to, of course, and if yours does not bring in the kind you like, you can get one with a wider range. If you no longer hear well, change from music to reading or visual art; if you no longer see well, turn to music.

If there is nothing at all that you can go back to, learn something new. Excellent adult-education classes are available in many cities, and programs on public television teach painting, sculpture, needlework, and other crafts. From other television programs you can learn how to please a gourmet and become a gourmet to be pleased, what kinds of plants will grow in your space, and how to have the green thumb you may have thought you never had. (In the absence of a sunny window, you can use a special kind of artificial light.) If you have never done things of that sort, you are to be envied for having so many still to explore. Pets are interesting. A bird or a few goldfish in a bowl need little care and can be taken to a neighbor's when you are away. A more sophisticated biological world—for example, an ant colony—can be fascinating. A cat or dog is more trouble but, of course, offers more companionship.

Try living a rather different kind of daily life. Just for a week or two experiment with different newspapers or magazines and different kinds of books. Watch different television programs and listen to different radio stations. See different people by going to different places. Perhaps you will find new things to do, and in addition, the novelty itself may be worthwhile. You may even become an enthusiastic explorer.

Gambling

Many old people turn to gambling for a touch of excitement. An evening of bingo, a weekly ticket in a state lottery or numbers game, an occasional bet on the horses—these are certainly the kinds of things people enjoy; and some kind of gambling has always been characteristic of the leisure class, to which you now in a sense belong.

Gambling adds to the enjoyment of life, however, only if you stay within your means, placing only the bets you can afford to lose. Look closely at the odds. State lotteries are a bad bet. They pay back only a ridiculously small part of the money they collect. The odds at horse racing are somewhat better. Roulette takes only a small amount for the house, and the house takes nothing when you play cards or organize a football pool with friends.

People do not gamble because they win. In the long run they almost always lose. (If the profits went to the betters, nobody would bother to set up bingo parlors, casinos, numbers games, horse races, or state lotteries.) Nevertheless, people gamble and enjoy the excitement, because of the unpredictability of the results. The same unpredictability made parcheesi, solitaire, and the high school football game exciting when you were young.

There are safer ways of enjoying unpredictable consequences. Baseball, football, basketball, hockey, golf, and other sports hold their television audiences to an extent that has amazed many people, and they do so just because the pay-offs are unpredictable. A football game is like a slot machine. A gain of five yards is two cherries; a first down, three oranges; the touchdown that wins the game, the jackpot. And, of course, games are more exciting if you have a bit of money riding on the outcome.

If you have never watched sports on television, you may be puzzled by the absorption of those who do—and perhaps a little contemptuous of those who so passionately care whether a ball goes out of the park, between the goal posts, through a basket, or into a hole. But should you not envy them? Or join them? Very often we answer a question of that sort by saying, "I don't think I would like it." But what you first see on the screen is not what the devotees are seeing. They know the game and the importance of every move. So will you if you listen to a good announcer for a few hours and discover what is really going on. You can then begin to enjoy the game and share the excitement of those who are held by its unpredictable consequences.

You may also be a little contemptuous of those who watch soap operas. If you have never done so, a short sample will not mean much, but remember, again, that you are not seeing what those who follow a serial see. Only when you have watched a number of episodes will you know what is happening and be prepared for the occasional exciting surprise. The novels of Dickens, Trollope, and others were first published as serials, and if you had sampled one episode halfway through *David Copperfield,* you would probably not have liked it either.

The difference between cheap and good literature is largely a difference in the distribution of exciting events. A comic strip provides a laugh at the end of every four frames, and in cheap literature something moderately interesting happens on almost every page. When you have learned to enjoy good literature, you read longer passages that are not in themselves interesting for the sake of the rare but much more moving events for which you are then prepared. It does not take any time to discover whether you will like a comic strip or cheap literature, but give yourself time to learn to enjoy good literature, art, and music. They are called good for good reasons.

CHAPTER 8

Getting Along with People

"The most dangerous weakness of old people who have been amiable," said La Rochefoucauld, "is to forget that they are no longer so." That is only a special case of the classical problem of aging: we do what we learned to do when we were younger and more successful. Just as our ability to see and hear, to move quickly and skillfully, and to think clearly may have diminished, so also our relations with other people may have deteriorated. This change is all the more dangerous, as La Rochefoucauld pointed out, because we are less likely to be aware of it.

We must ask, however, whether the change is primarily in ourselves or in the world in which we are living. Let us say that you were once a great conversationalist, but that now you do not easily think of things to say. Some of the change may be in the people you talk to, if they are no longer interested in what you say. And you may be interested in fewer things yourself because your world has grown smaller. Moreover, you more quickly forget. You read something in the morning paper that should interest a particular friend, but you forget to mention it when you have the chance. In such a case it is not always easy to replace memories with memoranda; you cannot very well carry a notebook of things to tell your friends when you see them. But you can certainly do something of that sort for the friends with whom you correspond.

Being a Good Companion

A change in your style of life may test your amiability. For example, one of the inconveniences of old age for you may be that you have had to stop driving a car. If you are lucky, others now drive you where you want to go. They may not continue to do so unless you learn to be a good passenger. Everyone complains about back-seat driving, and almost no one stops doing it. You may feel that you are merely being helpful when you point out that traffic is moving more quickly in another lane, that the stop light changed to green two seconds ago, or that another route is probably shorter, but your driver will not often thank you. You may not like the suggestion that, as a grateful passenger, you should put a piece of adhesive tape across your lips, but an imagined tape will help. Count the number of times you make suggestions during a ride of a particular length, and congratulate yourself as the number gradually decreases. To make some progress toward a more relaxed passengerhood, try imagining that you are riding in a bus, which goeth where it listeth.

Far worse, for you, than driving a car vocally is driving it silently. Back-seat driving is bad for the driver; silent driving is bad for you. You see another car approaching from an intersection and push both feet against the floorboards. The green light ahead will probably turn red before you reach it, and you either step on an imaginary accelerator or simply *wish* the car into a higher speed. You notice the physiological effect as a feeling of stress or tension. That stress is real—and dangerous. It is a classical example of the problem of aging: when you were a driver you kept your eyes steadily on the road for good reason, but what was formerly essential has become inappropriate; now you have an equally good reason to keep your eyes off the road.

And that is the way to solve the problems of both vocal and silent driving. *Stop looking at the road ahead.* Look at what you are passing. In the country, study the progress of the seasons, the different kinds of fields and wood lots, the clouds. In the city, study the architecture, the way people are dressed, what they seem to be doing. You will find yourself discovering much that is new about the old familiar places. When the passing scene palls, lower your eyes and think of something else. Learning to stop looking at the road may take you a long time, but you will be surprised at how easy it becomes, how much you enjoy what you see, and how much better you (and your companion!) will feel at the end of a journey.

Back-seat driving is only one example of a much broader complaint that is especially likely to be leveled against old people. As you gradually withdraw from the role of doer, you are likely to find it more and more tempting to tell others what to do and how to do it. Unwanted advice is seldom helpful, and it rarely makes the adviser a more valued companion.

Avoiding Embarrassment

Social amenities suffer when you have poor hearing or eyesight. Walking in a busy street you may not recognize acquaintances in time to say hello. Since not seeing is more forgivable than snubbing, you do better to avoid looking at the faces of the people you pass. If instead you say hello to everyone you may conceivably know, you run the risk of being taken for a campaigning politician. When you do meet a friend, be sure to look for the outstretched hand. When talking with a group of people in poor light, you may not be able to see who is speaking, and in an inattentive moment you may miss the fact that someone has addressed a remark especially to you. If you suffer from that kind of social mistake, you must follow conversations closely.

If you no longer enjoy some of the things you do with other people, you may have to take steps to stop doing them. Let us say that you accept an invitation to go with friends to a dark, noisy restaurant. You formerly liked to eat out with a group. But now you have trouble reading the menu; you cannot hear a word of what the person across the table is saying to you; and when your plate is removed, you find that you have pushed a messy bit of food onto the tablecloth. If this

were your first visit to such a restaurant, you
would never go again. There is only one solution:
escape from the control exercised by the fun you
once had. When you receive an invitation, think
of the probable consequences of accepting it.
Limit yourself to the kinds of things you enjoy
doing *as you are now.* You may need to be firm
with well-meaning friends who forget that you do
not enjoy what they still enjoy.

Staying Friendly

If you are seeing fewer friends, either because
there *are* fewer or because seeing them is difficult,
you may find it worthwhile to contact old ones.
You probably have friends you have not heard
from for years who would be delighted to hear
from you. You can write to them, as in the old
days, if writing is not too much of a burden, or
you can telephone if the rates are low for the area
in question or you can afford long-distance
charges. With a tape recorder talk is cheap. Cassettes can be mailed like letters, and if popping
cassettes into and out of your recorder is not too
much trouble, you can stop listening to your
friend's recorded message long enough to make
comments of your own on another tape to be sent
in reply. (With two recorders you can carry on an

enjoyable conversation—listening and replying as you please, and never being interrupted!)

People who do not choose each other's companionship but are thrown together may find it hard to get along. Retirement may raise that problem even for a husband and wife because it greatly increases the amount of time they spend together. The wife often feels that her house has been invaded by someone who does not belong there. But living comfortably with another person is better than living alone, and anything that can be done to make it possible is worth doing. If you are now living alone, trying to live with another person may take a bit of courage, but it can be worthwhile, particularly if the ground rules are carefully specified. Standards have changed, and it is no longer unusual for an old man and an old woman to live together without benefit of clergy. Loss of Social Security benefits is only one of the reasons why they may choose not to marry. It is now quite acceptable to advertise for friends: "Widower, late sixties, into Zen Buddhism, Bartók, world government, seeks lively correspondent, similar interests. Object: cohabitation."

Getting Along with Younger People

Jonathan Swift resolved that when he "came to be old," he would not "keep young company unless they really desire it." It is good advice and, once again, a recognition of our basic problem: we do what we learned to do when we were younger. The world was younger then too. The things we talk about now are no longer the latest things. Our jokes are no longer fresh. Our in phrases are now out. Unless we spend a great deal of time with young people, we cannot successfully imitate them. We do better to accept the date on the birth certificate and act our age. We shall then make fewer mistakes with both young and old.

Swift also resolved "not to be over severe with young people but give allowances for their youthful follies and weaknesses." It is curious that every generation should think that the next one is "going to the dogs." Obviously, this cannot be true; the world has survived for too many generations. You will probably not change young people much by criticizing, and you will certainly not make yourself a better companion by doing so.

You will necessarily impose some limitations upon your younger associates. In playing a game like tennis or golf or simply taking a walk with young people, you will obviously hold them back. Neither you nor your companions will fully enjoy the activity. The limitations may not be as obvious in other areas, but perhaps it is better to resolve:

> . . . Let me not live, . . .
> After my flame lacks oil, to be the snuff
> Of younger spirits.[1]

A friend we have not seen for a long time usually seems to have changed more than the people we see every day. We ourselves are one of the people we see every day and, perhaps fortunately, are often not aware of how much we have changed. Slight disfigurements—facial hair, an unsightly mole—can appear so slowly that we scarcely notice them. But others notice them—young people especially—and we are more likely to be acceptable company if we do whatever we can to make them less disturbing. They are a sign of age, but not the kind that we should proudly flaunt. It may help to have a photograph taken in unflattering light. Compared with the face we see every day in the mirror, a photograph may be like the friend we have not seen for a long time.

---

[1]*All's Well That Ends Well.*

Getting Along with Children

When the children you must get along with are your own, hard questions often have to be answered. Do you live with or near them, or they with you? Improved economic conditions have contributed to the demise of the large family that included some grandparents and an uncle and aunt or two. If you have resisted this trend and are still living with your children, problems may arise. We seldom speak to a spouse, parent, child, or sibling with the manner and tone of voice we adopt when speaking with casual acquaintances. If you live with your children, try thinking of them as friends.

Swift must have seen old people fawning over children. When he came to be old, he said, he would "not . . . be fond of children, or let them come near me hardly." Young children today freely show how they feel, and you will learn soon enough whether they or their parents like what you do. But if children enjoy your company, they can be a pleasure, and taking care of them can be one of the uses of grandparents as well as a part-time occupation for old people who need money or something to do.

If it has been a long time since you were with children, do not expect them to like you if you simply "come as you are." They have keen noses, eyes, and ears, and they may find old people very different from the people they most often see. They will need time to learn to like you, and you may need to help them do so. Some of the better programs on public television can serve as useful models, and you have an advantage over Mr. Rogers in that you and the children can do things together. A small repertoire of string figures, paper foldings, and magic tricks, carefully husbanded, will confer status. Jokes, verses, and conundrums will spice a youthful conversation. Guessing games and simple card games help. Good stories are never told often enough for the very young. If possible, advance to instruction—teach children simple poems or songs. Above all, conserve your stock; when children are enjoying themselves by themselves, leave them alone. (The world changes. Be prepared for surprises when you see what children are up to these days.)

CHAPTER 9

Feeling Better

Keeping in better touch with the world, suffering less from forgetfulness and from not thinking clearly, working and spending your time in more interesting ways, living in pleasanter surroundings, and enjoying yourself more with your friends—these are things you *do*. What about the things you *feel?* Although it has been said that old people do not have strong feelings, they have never lacked a reputation for resentment, jealousy, fear, depression, and other feelings that we should all rather be without. What about the feelings we enjoy? Is there some reason why they are out of reach of old people?

If you went to your doctor and told him that you were not feeling well, you would be surprised if he merely said "Feel better" and sent you home. Yet that is the way many people treat other kinds of feelings. If you tell your friends that you are depressed, they are likely to say "Cheer up." If on the way to the airport you talk about the bad flying weather, you may be told, "Don't worry." Possibly you will be more cheerful or less worried because someone cares enough about you to say "Cheer up" or "Don't worry," but these are not the kind of orders you can obey. Like our title, "Enjoy Old Age," they are wishes. And not very helpful wishes unless something is done to make them come true.

Instead of telling you simply to feel better, your doctor will tell you to get more exercise, to cut down on saturated fats, to get a prescription filled and take a pill so many times a day. These are things to do rather than feel, but when you have done them you will probably feel better. It is not *how* you feel that matters so much as *what* you feel. Your doctor has told you how to have a body that feels better. Something of the sort holds for other kinds of feelings. When we first said "Enjoy old age," you may have felt like replying "I will if you can make old age enjoyable." And, like the doctor, we must go beyond telling you how to feel. We must tell you how to change what is felt.

It could be said that the doctor goes directly to

the feeling when he gives you a drug that makes you feel better even when ill. Americans take billions of pills every year to feel better about their lives even when their lives remain wretched. For the same reason, and without a doctor's help, they turn to alcohol, marijuana, cocaine, and heroin. You are, of course, free to do so, but changing what you feel rather than how you feel is a better policy. Just as aspirin may cure a headache without curing the condition responsible for it, so drugs that make you feel better can keep you from attacking the condition that makes you feel bad. You can feel better by improving what you feel.

Depression is a good example. It is said to be the most prevalent mental-health disorder for people over sixty-five. If your depression is due to a physical illness, you must get treatment for that illness, but you may also feel depressed, as we have seen, simply because you can no longer do many of the things you have enjoyed. Perhaps you have liked talking to people but now there is no one to talk to. Perhaps you have enjoyed the countryside but are now cooped up in the city. Finding someone to talk to or some way of getting to the countryside will be better than remaining alone in the city taking Valium.

In earlier chapters we might have noted some of the feelings associated with the various things you do or fail to do—feelings that could often be changed by doing things in a different way. If you do not get around easily in the world in which you live (chapter 3), you may feel bewildered or lost; you will feel better if you find new ways of keeping in touch with that world or if you create a world that is less troublesome. If you forget things and do not think very clearly (chapters 4 and 5), you may suffer embarrassment or feel foolish. You will not be helped by someone who says "Don't be stupid"; you must find or create a world in which you can act in a more sensible way. If you have nothing to do (chapters 6 and 7), you may feel listless and depressed, but you cannot simply resolve to feel active and cheerful; you must find interesting things to do. If you do not make friends easily (chapter 8), you may feel lonely or unwanted, but you cannot simply resolve to be more friendly. The obvious solution is to become a more likable person or find friends who like you as you are. In all these examples you change your feelings by changing what is felt. You do so, however, only by changing the conditions responsible for what is felt.

Old people are often also troubled by feelings that are not so closely associated with the conditions we have surveyed. Here are a few samples:

Anger

One kind of anger comes from failure. You find yourself angry at the needle you cannot thread or the faucet that keeps dripping no matter how tight you close it. The anger is pointless; it does not put the thread through the needle or stop the dripping. You would do better to find a needle-threader or a bigger needle and to put a new washer in the faucet. These are painfully obvious suggestions, but the principle they represent is far from obvious. Don't wrestle with your anger. Control it by controlling its cause. If you are mad at your landlord, don't try to like him. Clear up the issue between you and him, or move out. (A tranquilizer will help, but it will also keep you from solving the problem in a better way.) If you find that you are angry more often than you used to be, perhaps the reason is that your problems are harder to solve. You are more likely to solve them if you recognize their source—not the angry disposition of an old person, but the world in which that old person lives.

Old people are sometimes envious or resentful of the young because they enjoy themselves in ways which used to be forbidden. It is a little late for old people to enjoy the new privileges of the young; they must find ways to discover and enjoy the privileges of being old. When they do so, they may even find that young people will envy them for some of the perquisites of age.

Sexual Love

The sexual activity that is so explicitly described in novels and portrayed in films almost always involves young people. A passionate love scene between two people much beyond middle age would probably be called impossible or ridiculous. It would not excite readers or audiences because they would find it hard to believe in the excitement of the participants. The golden years are supposed to be golden in other ways.

It is perhaps only natural that sexual activity in old people should be relatively infrequent. There are no genetic consequences that would select for an inclination to be sexually active in women who can no longer bear children, and men have always been in oversupply as procreative agents. Nevertheless, we cannot accept as always true the common belief represented in Hamlet's statement to his mother about her marriage to his uncle:

> You cannot call it love; for at your age
> The hey-day in the blood is tame, it's humble,
> And waits upon the judgment.

Sex is not always something that old people must leave to considered judgment.

Some help may be needed. The theologian Paul Tillich argued that pornography could be justified on the grounds that it extended sexuality into old age. After all, when life is no longer very exciting, we read exciting books and watch exciting movies and plays, and when life is no longer very amusing, we read funny books and watch funny movies and plays. When our life is no longer very erotic, should we not read erotic books and watch erotic movies and plays? We not only identify with the people we read about or watch, we respond in our own way to what they respond to. We are excited because others are excited and because of what they are excited about. We laugh with them and at the things they laugh at, and we can share their sexual excitement and be excited sexually by the things that excite them. Of course we are not all excited, amused, or aroused by the same things. If we have lost an interest in sex, we may claim the advantage that we are less driven by strong passion and hence less likely to get into trouble.

Old people are evidently rather more successful in maintaining affectionate relationships than young ones. When a young couple is divorced, almost no one pays any attention. The divorce of an old couple makes the newspapers, with a story emphasizing the number of years the marriage lasted.

It is too bad that affectionate relations between people of different ages are viewed uneasily. It is hard to see what is wrong with love between people of different ages, provided it is mutual. Everyone thinks the love of parents for their children and of children for their parents is highly commendable—as long as it is not sexual love. To be sure, close relations between persons of different ages are often due to other kinds of consequences, often financial, but that should not be allowed to generate guilt by association.

Fear

Old people have many things to be afraid of. Understandably, illness is one of them. As someone has said, when there is a possibility that you will be arrested, every knock on the door is an alarm. An illness is a knock on the door. Even trivial symptoms are frightening. Forgetting a familiar name may look like the beginning of senility. (Actually only from 2 to 6 percent of people over sixty-five suffer from senile dementia.) Fear is particularly dangerous if you are afraid to find out whether you are really ill. You can eliminate the fear only by getting a diagnosis and, if neces-

sary, doing something about it. Much the same
thing may be said of financial worries. Finding
out whether you have enough money for your
present way of life or should live more cheaply is
better than living as you now live while worrying
about the future.

Suspicion

When you are hard of hearing, you can easily
imagine that others are talking about you. When
you can no longer see well, you can easily suppose
that someone is smiling at a mistake you have
made. Daily life may be puzzling. The check pre-
sented by the waiter seems to have too many
items on it, but it is hard to see, and to examine
it closely would attract attention. Clerks can take
advantage of you if you accidentally pay too much
("Was that a ten-dollar bill or a twenty that I
gave you?"). No one has yet marketed a drug to
make you feel less suspicious. In any case you
would be suspicious about taking it. It would
make you dangerously vulnerable to everyone.

Some kind of clarification of your life is an
obvious solution. Insist on moving at your own
pace. You are quite right to be suspicious of the
fast talker. Never trust your memory. If you reduce the number of occasions on which people

can take advantage of you, you will be less bothered by suspicion. (And the more you enjoy your life, the less there will be for others to talk about behind your back.)

Helplessness

Loss of control of one's bodily functions can be humiliating, and all possible precautions should be taken. Other embarrassments may be residues of an early training that no longer applies. You were once told not to dawdle; now other people have to wait for you as you move more slowly. You were once told not to be impolite or snobbish; now you find that you have not heard someone speak to you or have failed to take the hand extended toward you. You were taught to do your share; now you cannot do as much as others. But the old punitive sanctions no longer apply, and there is no reason why you should suffer from them. Flaunt your imperfections if necessary, but in any case accept them as a degree of helplessness that should be tolerated by everyone.

Some questions are not easy to answer. At what point should you gracefully accept a seat on the bus, or assistance in carrying your packages, or an arm to be taken as you cross the street? How should you deal with the condescending manner of a person giving you instructions or information in detail that would be suitable for a ten-year-old child? You face much the same problem in the fulsome encouragement of well-meaning friends who sound like kindergarten teachers with their "But that is very *good!*" (Of course, instead of adding, "You are really growing up!" they next say, "You are not really getting old!") There is not much you can do. Perhaps a bit of true humility is the answer to humiliation.

In all these examples, what people feel is the by-product of what they do and of the circumstances under which they do it. Instead of trying to feel differently by some act of will, you do better to change what is felt by changing the circumstances responsible for it.

CHAPTER 10

"A Necessary End"– The Fear of Death

People sometimes reconcile themselves to an unhappy old age with the quip that "it is better than the alternative." In *Measure for Measure*, Shakespeare put it this way:

> The weariest and most loathed worldly life
> That age, ache, penury, and imprisonment
> Can lay on nature, is a paradise
> To what we fear of death.

It is doubtful, however, that fearing death makes life any more enjoyable.

Much of the problem is the uncertainty. Our own death is not one of the things we learn about from experience. We may have seen others die, but that is a different thing. We have also heard or read what other people say about death, but their information is no better than ours.

Religions have tried to resolve the uncertainty in many ways. In some, like Buddhism, death is a time of great enlightenment. In others, like Judaism, it is simply an end, after which one survives, if at all, only in honored memory. In still others, like Christianity, it is a time for judgment and the assignment of punishments and rewards in another world. The fear varies accordingly. It is said that Zen Buddhism made the samurai a great warrior because it freed him from any fear of death. Christians who are sure of their future in another world may share that freedom, but those who are not sure, either of their future or of the truth of what they have been told, may remain afraid.

If your religion or philosophy has given you an answer, nothing we say here will matter. Nevertheless, to the extent that a fear of death can seriously affect the enjoyment of life, some remarks may be in order.

The biology of death is simple enough. The human body is largely self-renewing and lasts a remarkably long time, but it nevertheless plays a relatively brief part in the evolution of the species. As far as the species is concerned, individuals need to live only through the years in which they bear and possibly care for their young. After that they are useless—and worse than useless if they occupy space and consume goods that are needed by those who are still reproducing.

A different role emerged when the human species evolved to the point at which property was shared and information was passed from one individual to another. Those who were no longer reproductive could then support, advise, teach, and otherwise help those who were still reproductive. The role of the individual began to be much more important in the evolution of a culture than of the species. However, the advantages to the culture have not been felt long enough to bring about the kind of genetic change that would extend life.

Bodies wear out, and even the most enjoyable old age must come to an end. Before it does, a few practical steps can be taken. A properly executed will can give you the satisfaction of knowing that your possessions will go to the right people. You can extend the life of at least a small part of you by arranging for any organs that are still in good condition to be put to use in someone else's body.

When that has been done, it is probably better not to think about death. As Franklin Delano Roosevelt did not exactly say, the only thing we have to fear about death is that the fear of death will make it impossible to enjoy our lives. If after death you are to be either rewarded or punished according to what you have done in this life, and if you have no clear assurance of which it will be, you are perhaps well cautioned to "remember that you will die" *(memento mori)* even though you will then probably enjoy this life less. If on the other hand you accept the word of Ecclesiastes that there is "no better thing under the sun, than to eat, and to drink, and to be merry," you may wish to leave the question of death to be answered only when necessary.

> . . . death, a necessary end,
> Will come when it will come.[1]

There are strategies that may help. What arouses fear is not death itself, but the act of talking and thinking about it, and that can be stopped. When you are bored with a conversation, you change the subject. When you are sick of the tune you are humming, you hum a different tune. Making the change is easier if the new subject is more interesting than the old or the new tune pleasanter. In the same way, you can turn your attention away from death. Unfortunately, the very independence now enjoyed by old people has had the effect of throwing them

[1] *Julius Caesar.*

together with other old people. When grandparents lived with or near their children and grandchildren, they constantly saw younger people living younger lives. Now, in Florida or California or in nursing homes, they are much more likely to see only other old people, and health and death are favorite topics of conversation. Anything you can do to spend part of your time with younger people, together with a strong resolution to avoid talking about death with old people, will be worthwhile.

We brood about death most when we have nothing else to do. We brood much less when watching an exciting television program or doing something in which we are deeply interested. Everything we do to make old age more enjoyable reduces the time we spend in fearing death. The more reason we have to pay attention to life, the less we have to pay attention to death. (Please note that we have made this chapter mercifully short.)

Getting Out of the Way

When you find it truly impossible to enjoy your life, you pass out of range of this book. You face a problem that Western cultures have never solved. Few of us want to be a burden to others or to go on living in pain, but if we can no longer take care of ourselves or enjoy good health, there is little we can do. With Whitman we may look to the "delicious nearby freedom of death," but only looking is legal. Many people have earnestly wanted to die—for their own sake or the sake of others—but society has not made dying easy. It may even oppose the use of drugs, such as heroin, that not only kill the pain of those terminally ill but make them feel better in possibly the only remaining way. Society opposes suicide, often for religious reasons, even though many respected old people have chosen that way out. Helping people commit suicide, even describing ways in which it can be done painlessly, is usually illegal. (In England, a *Guide to Self-Deliverance* was made available by a society interested in euthanasia, but only to members of three months' standing and over twenty-five years of age, and they were cautioned not to lend it to others. A similar book in France created a furor.) We dispose of an old dog in a way that is called humane —ironically, since it is denied to human beings. Many old people, living in pain or as a burden to others, would be glad to be put to death caninely. About all that can be done, and that with doubtful effect, is to leave a living will instructing those who are caring for you not to take any unusual measures to keep you alive.

CHAPTER 11

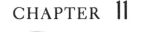

Playing Old Person

All the world's a stage, and you are not the first to play the part of Old Person. The audience has seen the play thousands of times and knows your lines better than you do. The role you are expected to play is not flattering. The Old Persons who have walked the boards before you have been crotchety, stingy, boastful, boring, demanding, and arrogant. They have complained of their illnesses and many other things. You may be surprised at how easy it is to play the part that way. The audience expects such a performance and, like a child listening to a bedtime story, will not tolerate many changes. And just as an audience will laugh at everything a great comedian says, so it will interpret your slightest gesture as the skillful portrayal of a familiar, and usually unpleasant, character.

It would be wrong to conclude that the role you play must represent the real you. Young people show the same traits as old people when they are exposed to the same circumstances, and if certain traits seem especially to characterize the old, that is because for the old the circumstances giving rise to them are more frequent and compelling. The point is important for practical reasons. If the traits of stinginess, boastfulness, and so on are inborn and simply mature as people grow older, not much can be done about them; if their frequent presence can be traced to special features of the world of old people, the problem is easier to solve. If you are not displaying your character, but are merely being a good character actor, you may play a different role as convincingly under different circumstances.

A Few Examples

Old people are, indeed, often stingy. In general they probably tip less than younger people, complain more about prices, give cheaper gifts. But they are also probably not earning as much as they must spend, and what they have saved or are receiving as Social Security is shrinking with inflation. They do not find it easy to go on paying more and more for the same food at the supermarket or more rent for the same apartment. Another reason for stinginess applies as well to the affluent. The fairness of a price is one of the things old people learned when they were young. An action that is now called stingy may not have been stingy when it first became habitual. Just as old people continue to use outmoded expressions and dress in slightly outmoded ways, so they continue to give a quarter to the cloakroom attendant when others are giving a dollar. If you would play the role of Old Person in modern dress, you must learn new lines and new stage business.

Old people are often boring. For one thing, they talk too much about the old days. When the old and the people they talked to were both young, those were the new days, and talk about them was talk about current events. Now, what the old talk about seems to their young audiences to be ancient history. Unless you are an exceptional storyteller, your young friends will not find history as interesting as you do. Perhaps you should set a date. Unless asked to do so, do not talk about personal experiences of more than a decade ago.

Old people are boring also because they share fewer interests with the people they most often see. When they were young they chose most of their friends because of common experiences and interests. At work they talked with their associates about common problems. They joined organizations related to their special interests. But they lose most such opportunities to share interests when they retire and live with their children, or in special housing for the elderly, or in a warmer climate where their neighbors are chosen by real-estate agents. One solution is to look for people with whom mutually interesting things can be discussed.

Old people are also often boring because they tend to repeat themselves. (Swift resolved "not to tell the same story over and over to the same people.") Young people too repeat a good story when they find a new audience, but old people have told their good stories many more times and hence are all the more likely to tell them again to the same audience. And they are more likely to forget that they have already told them. When something reminds you of one of your favorite stories, play safe and ask whether you have told it before, and make it clear that you truly want to know.

It is easy to be converted into a bore by those who, showing due respect for your age, give you a false report of success. Their nods and smiles encourage you to go on. They would walk out on you if you were on a real stage, but they politely hear you out. You will not have as large an audience at the next performance. The wedding guest would no doubt have been happy to meet the Ancient Mariner again, but we do not all have Coleridge's gifts. Courtesy and respect for old age also contribute to another boring trait—long-windedness. The young will let you run on. *Make allowances for the allowances that are made for you as an old person.*

Old people are boring when they talk about their illnesses. And so, very often, are young people. Operations and the latest medical advances are fascinating, but usually only to those who have profited from them. The longer you live the more of them you have to talk about. And there is another reason why the subject of illness so often comes up. People talk about the weather not because it is often important but because it is there when an embarrassing pause must be filled. The illnesses of old people are always, and often painfully, available in that kind of emergency, and the greeting "How are you?" calls attention to them.

The best way to avoid talking about illness is, of course, not to be ill, but perhaps that is too much to ask. What is needed is a good reason *not* to talk about it. The heroism shown by those who do not complain of extreme pain may be worth emulating on a smaller scale. Can you be the

famous old person who *never* talks about aches
and pains? If so, you may find that you are not
only more highly honored but more often welcomed as good company.

It is often said that old people are braggarts.
They do not all resolve to

> . . . speak not like a dotard nor a fool,
> As under privilege of age to brag
> What I have done being young, or what would do
> Were I not old.[1]

The conspicuous imperfections of age are a
handy excuse for current failure, and it is easy for
old people to boast about past exploits because
they cannot be asked for a demonstration. A
more successful old age should be the solution—
unless, of course, you begin to boast too much
about your successful management of old age.

Old people are inclined to moralize. La Rochefoucauld pointed to one reason: "Old age con-
soles itself by giving good precepts for being un-
able to give bad examples." But there is also a
better reason. The mistake old people make is,
again, to continue to do things in outmoded ways.
When they were young they criticized to good
effect contemporaries who violated prevailing

[1]*Much Ado About Nothing.*

standards. Now, at least with the young, criticism based on these same standards has little or no effect, except to make the critic a less welcome companion. It is better to grant young people their own standards even if you continue to live by yours.

Summing Up

Misquotation is one of the prerogatives of old age, and we shall use it to summarize: it is not too late to convert old age into a land—

> Where people get old but not godly and grave,
> Where people get old but not crafty and wise,
> Where people get old but not bitter of tongue.[2]

You will feel that these comments are beside the point if you have welcomed old age as a time when you can *be* objectionable. More than one old person has exclaimed, "Thank God, I no longer have to be nice to people!" But that is a dangerous attitude. Young people took it with respect to their elders in the 1960s, and vagabonds and drifters have taken it with respect to everybody for thousands of years. A net gain is

[2]William Butler Yeats, *The Land of Heart's Desire* (roughly).

questionable. The culture of the sixties did not last, and not many people find Skid Row attractive. A few old people become successfully unpleasant "characters," but only by specializing in a particular kind of unpleasantness: they are crotchety but not stingy, or stingy but fun to be with for other reasons. Old age has its freedoms, but freedom from criticism is certainly not one of them.

To explain some of the unpleasant characteristics of old people in this way is not to exonerate them. Throughout this book we have been saying, as Shakespeare did not exactly put it, "The fault, dear Brutus, is not in our stars, *nor in ourselves,* that we are underlings. It is in the world in which we live." But we cannot therefore conclude that we should be exempt from criticism for our faults. That would be like saying that a juvenile delinquent should not be punished if the delinquency can be traced to a bad early environment. Criticism and other kinds of punishment are traditional ways of changing people, and they must remain in use until better ways are found— and that means until the environment of the young is made less destructive and the world of the old is greatly improved. We have looked at that world not to defend old people against criticism, but to see how it can be changed to make criticism unnecessary.

CHAPTER 12

A Great Performance –
"The Grandeur and
Exquisiteness of Old Age"

Someone, not Shakespeare, has said that life is a play with a badly written last act.[1] Perhaps that is why giving a really great performance is so hard. When played with skill the part of Old Person is marked by tranquility, wisdom, freedom, dignity, and a sense of humor. Almost everyone would like to play it that way, but few have the courage to try. Most would feel that they were badly cast. But are these the character traits of a few exceptional old people or the traits of ordinary people under exceptional circumstances? If the latter, can the circumstances not be changed in such a way that everyone who plays Old Person will give a better performance?

[1] It was Cicero.

Tranquility

Serenity, a rough synonym for *tranquility,* often refers to things—Gray's "gem of purest ray serene" is an example—but both words have long been used to describe a feeling or state of mind. However, the essential condition to which they refer lies outside the person. The world must be tranquil before the majority of old people can enjoy tranquility. A tranquil world will not be one in which they do not need to do anything. They will do less, but still enjoy it. Old age, as Emerson said, is a time to take in sail; but it is not a time to be wholly adrift.

Tranquility is sometimes thought of as a state in which old people live quiet lives within themselves—for example, by living on their memories. They certainly have more memories than the young to relive and more time to relive them, but whether they enjoy them depends upon what they are about. An old age devoted to remorse or regret cannot be very pleasant. As Leigh Hunt knew, happy episodes may be worth recalling:

> Say I'm weary, say I'm sad,
> Say that health and wealth have missed me,
> Say I'm growing old, but add,
> Jenny kissed me.

But remembering that sort of thing will not keep most old people busy very long.

Of course they will take pride in the ventures they have brought to a successful conclusion and in the warm friendships they have made. These are true *accomplishments*—things they have done. Unfortunately they are not things to do now. Urging old people to enjoy themselves by remembering the good life they have lived is rather like trying to help a depressed young man by saying, "Look at all the things you have going for you—a loving wife, happy children, a pleasant home, no financial worries." The trouble is that he has already achieved them. What he needs is something to do now. Trying to be happier by "recollecting in tranquility" your happier days is rather like trying to "hold a fire in [your] hand / By thinking on the frosty Caucasus." Alas, "the apprehension of the good / Gives but the greater feeling to the worse."[2]

Being quietly inactive may solve some problems, but doing absolutely nothing is rather like falling asleep when you are freezing to death; you will survive only if you find some way to remain active. Perhaps it is only very late in life that old people should specialize in tranquility.

[2]*Richard II.*

Wisdom

Not everyone goes early to bed and is early to rise, but almost everyone wants to be healthy, wealthy, and wise. We have left health and wealth to others. What can we say about wisdom? Certainly it is one of the qualities most often admired in old people, and in part just because they are old. They have been around a long time. They were "not born yesterday." They are seasoned, aged in the wood. They "know the road." The name of the Roman governing body was *senatus*, from *senex*, meaning "old," and many religions speak of those who hold important positions as "elders." The aldermen you may have voted for were once called eldermen.

Unfortunately, technological progress has robbed everyone, old and young alike, of the chance to serve as a repository of wisdom. In Plato's *Phaedrus*, Thamus complains of the invention of the alphabet. Henceforth, he says, people will seem to know things that they have only read about. The human race would not have gone very far if it had confined itself to personal knowledge, but it has, so to speak, moved knowledge almost completely out of heads and into books—and now, of course, into computers. Before the invention of writing, and then of printing, knowledge was transmitted orally, and mainly from old to young, but that has changed. Young people no longer turn to old artisans to learn their trade; they go to technical schools or agricultural colleges. They no longer listen to troubadours to learn the history of their race or nation; they read history. The sacred words of religion, once chanted by holy men, are now found in "scripture"—scrolls and bibles, pre- or post-Gutenberg. People are needed only when they possess the kind of knowledge that cannot yet be transmitted through books. We go to a doctor rather than a book when we are ill, to a violinist to study the violin, to a painter to study painting, to a coach to learn a sport. Some old people, too, are specialists in fields in which books have not wholly taken over.

Your grandchildren will probably not ask for your advice about choosing an occupation; they will talk with educational or career counselors. They may not even ask you what life was like when you were young; the curious old telephones, the old cars that were started with a crank, the funny clothes people wore, the absurd ways they danced—all these can be seen on late-night television. Perhaps you can recount a bit of family lore or some community history that has not been put into print, but the number of your listeners will be small.

The wisdom that is valued most in old people concerns old age itself. If you are really enjoying your life in spite of imperfections, you may find yourself an authority. People will come to you to learn your secret, and you would be churlish not to divulge it.

Freedom

Old age has been acclaimed as a liberation. Old people are said to be free from the strong passions that caused so much trouble when they were young and from the old compelling responsibilities and ambitions. But too much freedom of that sort can be dangerous. Cicero warned against relinquishing too many of your prerogatives: "Old age is honored only on condition that it defends itself, maintains its rights, is subservient to no one, and to its last breath rules over its own domain." King Lear discovered the essential mistake. Turn your kingdom over to your children and you may find yourself out in the cold. Something of the sort is often the fate of rich people who free themselves of responsibilities by turning their fortunes over to their children or to foundations; of businessmen who turn control of their companies over to younger people; of political figures who retire in favor of new blood; and of scientists, artists, composers, and writers who leave further work in their fields to others. They may not be as shabbily treated as Lear, but they may be surprised at the speed with which they are forgotten.

Old age nevertheless can be enjoyed as a time when one is relatively free of many responsibilities, strong emotions, and overriding ambition.

Dignity

The general who keeps a proper demeanor as he rides in a jeep over rough terrain, and the queen who shows no sign that she feels the champagne a careless servant has spilled down her neck, are admired for maintaining their dignity. Certain ultimate consequences have taken precedence over temporary distractions. Old people are, in a sense, always riding in bouncing jeeps and having things spilled on them. Some succeed in maintaining their dignity.

Looking old is often felt to be one of the indignities of age. If you were once attractive, you will remember the time when people (particularly those of the opposite sex) began to pass you on the street without a second look. So it is not surprising that old people often try to look younger than they are. But trying to look younger simply makes it all the harder to face the truth when you unquestionably look old. Looking younger is at least generally safe, but *acting* younger is dangerous. Trying to get on a bus with the light step of someone ten years younger can mean more than a loss of dignity. In old age, someone has said, some of the pleasures of youth can be enjoyed only on pain of death.

If you are now quite obviously old, you do best to look attractively old. If you have turned to a wig or hairpiece, choose one that looks like the hair of a person your age. After all, gray or white hair is distinguished and goes with any color of dress or necktie. Teeth make a difference and orthodontia is not just for adolescents. A good figure becomes more and more a matter of posture and you can usually do something about that. Arthritis may force you to stoop, but stooping is often only a matter of weak muscles. Shoulders can be straightened to some extent, and what begins as frequent deliberate straightening may eventually become automatic.

We are flattered when we are told that we look young, and all the more so the older we are. It was not always thus. When we were fourteen, we were probably delighted to be taken for sixteen, and when sixteen for eighteen, but somewhere in the early twenties the direction changed. When we were twenty-five, we were not likely to be flattered if taken for thirty, or when sixty for seventy. If you really enjoy your age, you may agree that to be pleased when judged younger is disloyal. "You don't look your age!" is meant as a compliment, but the proper reply is, "This is the way a person my age looks." Trying to look younger seldom succeeds. There is good reason to come out of the closet and look, act, and tell your age. You will be maintaining your dignity when you do so.

A Sense of Humor

The victims of joke-shop novelties are led to do things that have unexpected consequences. The cigarette lighter falls apart when they operate it; the candle they blow out relights, and relights again when they blow it out again. This kind of trick is not very funny, but it is the kind the world plays on old people. In a dimly lit restaurant you go on talking, unaware that your friend has left the table to go to the salad bar. You join in a conversation only to find that you have completely misunderstood what it was about. Others find your errors amusing. Can you be amused too?

We have all known people who seem to lack any sign of a sense of humor (of course, if we ourselves lack it, we shall not have noticed its absence), and we have all known people for whom life is little more than a perpetual joke. Is a sense of humor a genetic trait or a product of early experience? A more relevant question is whether anything can be done to acquire one late in life. We come home after a long day when everything has gone wrong, and we tell our husband or wife about it in either a string of complaints or a string of can-you-believe-it absurdities. There is a great difference in the result. As we complain, things are still going wrong, but the humor of the absurd brings the bad day to a pleasant end.

It has often been pointed out that the things we call funny are only milder versions of those we call unpleasant or painful. The pratfall of a young friend may be funny, but not if he breaks a hip. The quaint grammar of someone who speaks English as a second language is amusing; incomprehensible speech is annoying. One kind of witty remark is amusing until taken seriously; then it is an insult. The point at which something passes from funny to annoying depends upon the occasion. If you have been laughing, it is easier to go on laughing. That is why the audiences of supposedly funny television shows are put in a laughing mood before air time by a special entertainer who can use material not permitted on the air. Preparing people to find old age funny, is no doubt hard, but funny things can be added to their lives. Reading funny stories, watching funny shows on television, spending more time with one's funnier friends—all these are preferable to reading obituaries or stories about the tribulations of old age.

The real infirmities of old age must be taken seriously, but wherever possible the relief that comes from seeing the funny side should be cultivated. Perhaps you should start by practicing on episodes that are not too annoying. If you can succeed there, then with a little luck you may be able to move on to laugh at things you have found more distressing.

A Good Old Age

No matter how well the last act may have been rewritten, not everyone will play Old Person with panache. You may have to be satisfied with an adequate performance. In a script that plays well, you will enjoy a reasonable freedom from annoyances, a chance to do many of the things you like, and less reason to do things you do not like. A sense of humor will take care of some of the annoyances that remain. Much of this would be easier to accomplish if you had prepared for it when you were young, and you should have been more likely to prepare if you had looked forward to old age, not as something to be feared, but as a problem to be solved.

Applause for a Great Performance?

In chapter 11 we looked at some of the conditions that made the standard role of a crotchety, stingy, moralizing Old Person so easy to play. We did so, not to absolve old people of blame for such traits of character, but to see whether conditions could not be changed so that a better performance could be given. Suppose, now, that you are one of those who, because a better script has been written, are living a life marked by tranquility, wisdom, freedom, dignity, and a sense of humor. In attributing your performance to the script, are we not robbing you of personal credit? Can you have it both ways? If the fault, dear Brutus, is not in yourself but in the world in which you live, where is the credit found?

You need not worry. Audiences always hiss the villain and cheer the hero. You will be admired for your performance no matter how favorable the circumstances under which you give it. Admiration is one of the ways in which society encourages great performances, and it will go on applauding even if the part is so good that it is always beautifully played.

And if you yourself have constructed the world that permits you to live a tranquil, dignified, and enjoyable life, you will be doubly admired—not only for a great performance, but for writing a last act that plays so well.

Appendix

A Note on the Language in
Which This Book Is Written

The word *behavior* was first used five centuries ago, and since then it has taken on and discarded many special meanings. In *The Behavior of Organisms* (1938) I offered this definition: "Behavior is what an organism is *doing.*" That would be more helpful if the *Oxford English Dictionary* did not need six large three-column pages to record the history of the forms and significations of the word *do.* From the beginning, however, *do* has meant "achieve some kind of effect," and that is the central meaning of the word *behavior* in modern scientific usage. Whether innate or acquired, behavior is selected by its consequences. In natural selection the consequences are the contribution the behavior makes to the survival of the species. In operant conditioning the effective consequence is called a reinforcer. It strengthens the behavior in the sense of making it more likely to occur again in a similar setting. Operant conditioning is studied in the laboratory by arranging complex and subtle relations among setting, behavior, and consequence.

In reporting the results of such an analysis and in making a technical application of its principles to daily life, a technical vocabulary is needed. In showing how some of those principles can be used to solve a practical problem such as that of the enjoyment of old age, everyday English will usually suffice. We have not asked our readers to become specialists in the experimental analysis of behavior. For those who are curious, however, here are a few examples of the terms used in this book and roughly equivalent terms that would appear in a more rigorous analysis:

doing things = *behaving*

doing what one wants to do = *behaving in ways that have been positively reinforced*

doing what one has to do or must do = *behaving in ways that have been negatively reinforced*

doing what one likes to do = *behaving in ways that have momentary positively reinforcing consequences not necessarily related to ultimate consequences*

thinking about = *behaving (perhaps covertly) with respect to*
needing = *being deprived of*
enjoying = *being reinforced by*
knowing how to do something = *possessing a particular kind of effective behavior*
knowing about something = *possessing effective behavior under the control of a particular discriminative stimulus*

These are only rough equivalences. In typical sentences the terms on the left will not always neatly replace those on the right or vice versa. The same would have to be said of a similar list of equivalences in physics, chemistry, or biology.

Further equivalences can be found in B. F. Skinner, *Science and Human Behavior* (New York: Macmillan, 1953), and B. F. Skinner, *About Behaviorism* (New York: Alfred A. Knopf, 1974).

—B. F. S.